NATURALLY
STEFANIE

First published 2019
by Black & White Publishing Ltd,
Nautical House, 104 Commercial Street, Edinburgh, EH6 6NF

1 3 5 7 9 10 8 6 4 2   19 20 21 22

ISBN: 978 1 78530 279 4

All photography except on the pages listed below copyright © Euan Anderson
pp. 4, 12, 160 © Shutterstock
pp. 33, 35, 60, 67, 129, 135, 140, 232 © Stefanie Moir

A CIP catalogue record for this book is available from the British Library.

Design by creativelink.tv
Printed and bound in Spain by EstellaPrint

NATURALLY
STEFANIE

Simple plant-based recipes, workouts and daily rituals for a stronger, happier you

STEFANIE MOIR

BLACK & WHITE PUBLISHING

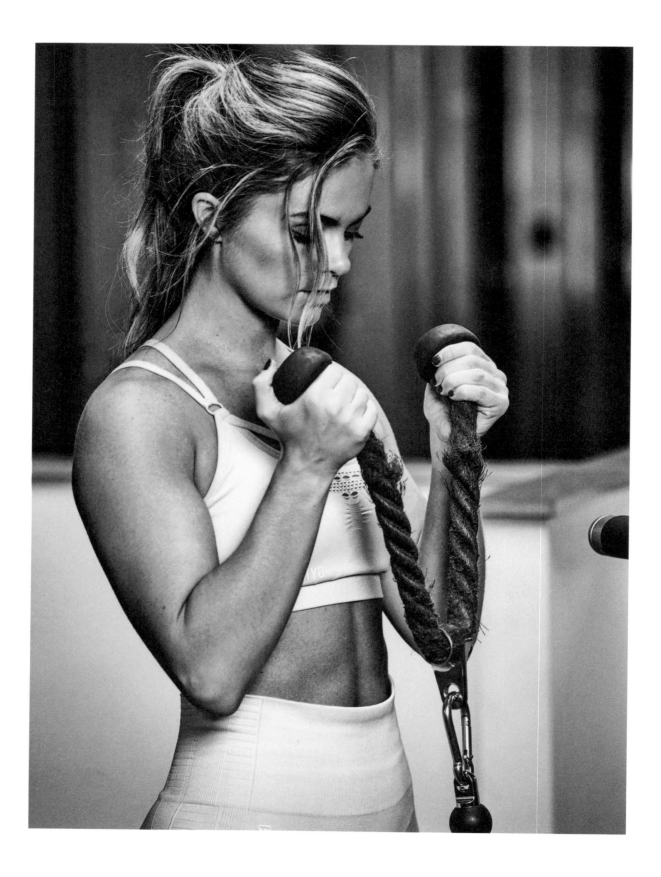

This book is for everyone who has followed and supported my journey so far, without you this wouldn't be possible.

And for my parents who have always supported me, shown me how to go after what I want and guided me the whole way, I love you.

———————————————————————

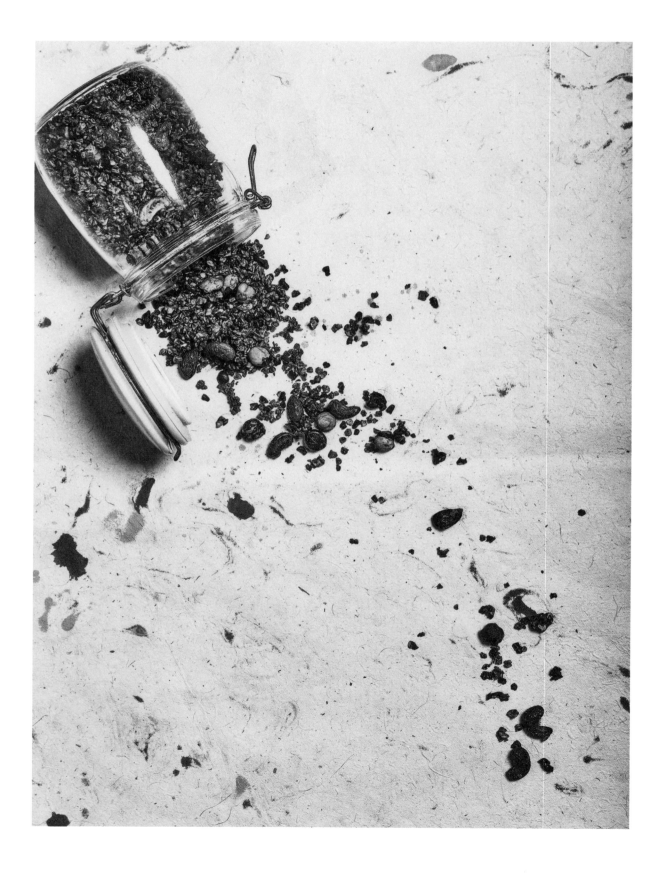

CONTENTS

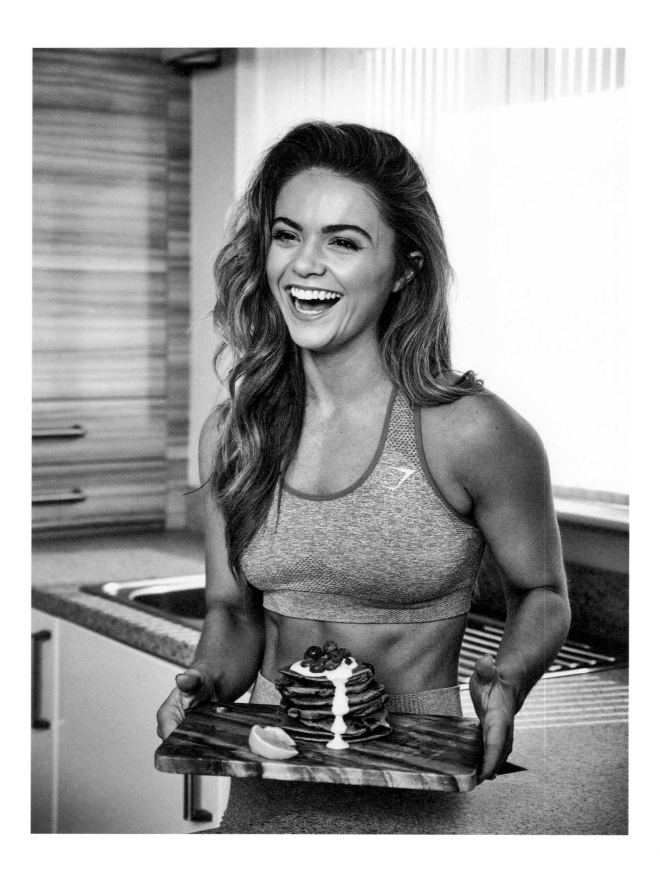

WELCOME

I'm Stefanie Moir, also known as Naturally Stefanie. I'm a vegan lifestyle blogger, avid gym goer and fitness website owner.

Welcome to my book! Since 2015, I have shared tips and tricks on how to become stronger, healthier and happier on my blog, YouTube channel and Instagram. It's been an inspiring journey – and I'm excited to combine all that I've learned into my first book.

You do not have to go plant-based overnight, nor do you have to go to the gym and have a six pack, to benefit from this book. My aim is to help you incorporate more plant-based meals into your life, and help you look and feel better along the way with workouts and routines aimed at people of all fitness levels.

A plant-based lifestyle is not a diet – nor is the gym the only place you can successfully, and happily, get fit. I do not advocate diets in any way shape or form. I believe in eating whole plant-based foods that are good for the body and soul and leave you feeling and looking your absolute best.

ABOUT ME

I grew up just outside of Glasgow. I have always loved sport and exercise, and was part of my local swimming club for over ten years. I went to university to study psychology in 2012 and it was around this time I moved on from swimming to weight training at the gym. I've been hooked ever since!

As I progressed with my training, I started looking into how to complement my new gym regime with a healthy diet – and found veganism. I soon found I was feeling better than ever before and started my blog, Naturally Stefanie, and my Instagram account, to document my vegan and weight training journey. My YouTube channel soon followed, and I began to share recipes and also to introduce more of myself and my lifestyle to my audience.

Over the four years of my degree studies, I fell more and more in love with fitness and nutrition. Once I'd graduated, I decided to put my heart and soul into my Naturally Stefanie brand. I would never have imagined I'd be where I am today, and I am so grateful for every opportunity that has presented itself over the last few years.

I now run my vegan fitness site, veganaesthetics.co.uk, which has built an amazing community of like-minded individuals from across the globe who have all been inspired to transform their health and wellbeing. By reading this book, you are now part of this community and I hope you'll be equally as inspired to start your journey towards a stronger, happier you!

MY HEALTH AND FITNESS JOURNEY

Many people join the gym, go for a week or two then give up. This doesn't mean that fitness and good health is inaccessible to them – maybe the gym is not for you, but exercise can be for everyone. I believe everyone can find a form of exercise they love – whether it be in the gym, the pool, at a dance class or out walking in nature.

I choose to work out around five or six days per week and focus on lifting weights. I am not a bodybuilder, nor do I plan to ever compete in any shape or form, but I do love to train and push my body with weights. I feel passionately about showing that a plant-based lifestyle is more than optimal for lean muscle building and overall exercise performance. The myth that you can't build muscle, or run fast, or out-swim your team mate on a plant-based, vegan lifestyle is just that – a myth.

When I first went vegan six years ago, the concern I received from my family and friends for my sporting performance and goals was at an all-time high. However, the last few years have debunked that myth (yes, I do get enough protein. Fancy that!), and living a plant-based lifestyle has only ever helped me achieve my fitness goals.

As a vegan, I make sure to eat a well-balanced diet, lots of fruits, vegetables, nuts, seeds, grains, legumes, beans and lots of homemade desserts. I am somewhat of a chocoholic – I think chocolate actually runs through my veins – and going vegan hasn't changed that.

CHANGING THE WAY YOU THINK ABOUT PLANTS

Eating plant-based meals is not about deprivation and restriction; you are not 'giving up' anything by eating more plant-based, you're switching it up instead. My main takeaway from plant-based living would be don't over complicate it, make healthy choices and cook the easy recipes in this book that you and your whole family will love. Don't be like 2013 me, trying to get all fancy following a horrendously complicated Pinterest recipe for cauliflower crust pizza and serving up slop on a plate. Stick to this book and you might make food you will actually enjoy eating . . .

I know from personal experience that the hardest part about making any kind of change to your life – whether it be your diet, working out, your job, your relationships – is the social aspect. Eating healthily or even using the word 'VEGAN' is still such a foreign concept to many that you might experience some concerns or backlash at first. People can often think that being vegan means you live off nothing but lettuce and telling someone you are going plant-based or vegan might seem daunting, but their reluctance to support you often comes from a place of concern – they think it is unhealthy when it can actually be quite the opposite.

Another thing you might worry you will struggle with as a vegan is eating out. However, veganism is now becoming more recognised and a large majority of restaurants now have vegan items on their menus; over the years I have watched many of my favourite restaurants actually bring out vegan menus. To make going out as easy as possible, perhaps check the menus of restaurants in advance to see they cater for your food choices – or if they'd be willing to tweak some of their meals to accommodate you – alternatively, cook some feasts from this book and invite everyone around to share it with you!

HOW TO USE THIS BOOK

Recipes account for much of this book – sweet and savoury breakfasts, nourish bowls, main meals, snacks and sweets – plenty to sink your teeth into (excuse the pun). When you start eating more healthy meals, planning and preparation is key. I would recommend picking out the recipes you like for the week and making a shopping list.

You can always make double the amount of a recipe so you have leftovers for the next day. I like to have my kitchen cupboards and fridge jam-packed with healthy food (and my sneaky stash of chocolate for good measure). You will have heard this a million times, but failing to prepare is preparing to fail, my friends. If you have healthy food, you will eat healthy food at home.

There are tips throughout this book to let you know what meals are great to make in bulk, which are good for pre- or post-workout and what recipes work well for big groups of friends and dinner parties. As mentioned, this book is not only aimed at vegans or those who wish to be 100 per cent vegan. It is for anyone who simply wants to introduce more healthy habits into their lifestyle. Whether you like to follow meat-free Mondays or simply want to spice up your weekly diet with some new recipes, there are options here that will work for everyone.

The final quarter of the book is packed with information regarding exercise, with a weekly plan showing how you can implement both a healthy diet and exercise into your week; and advice on how to take care of the soul, as well as the body. This could be the most important part of the book for you – so many of us are so busy with our day-to-day schedules that we forget to take time for ourselves and ensure we are giving ourselves some self-love.

It is my hope that anyone picking up *Naturally Stefanie* will be able to take even just one thing away from it, whether that is a change to their diet, starting up an exercise regime, paying closer attention to self-love – I wrote this book to be inclusive of everyone and with the aim to give something, no matter how small, to everyone who reads it.

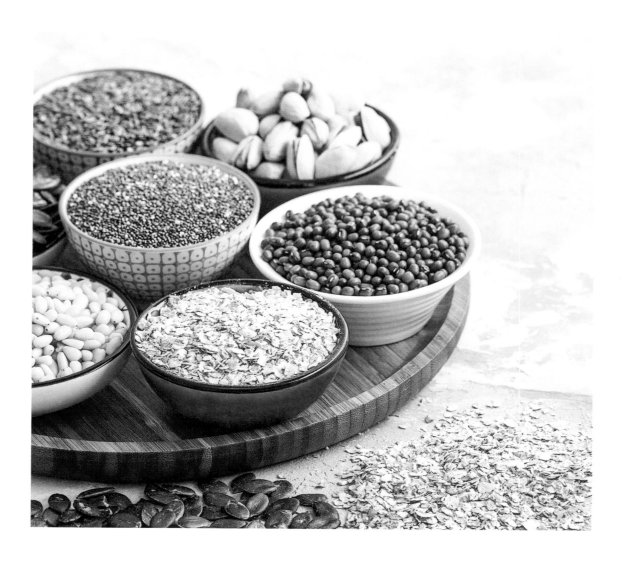

A NOTE ON PROTEIN

The recipes in *Naturally Stefanie* are protein-packed, nutrient-rich and full of fruits and veggies – covering all the essential vitamins and minerals your body needs to perform optimally. Please bear in mind that I am not a qualified nutritionist, and that everyone's bodies are different and need different things. A plant-based diet might not be suitable for everyone and if you are at all concerned about your health, I would recommend seeking medical guidance before embarking on a lifestyle change.

There are so many natural plant-based sources of protein available such as tofu, beans, lentils, and quinoa – all of which appear often in these recipes – which tick all the boxes to ensure you're getting your daily protein quota. Some plant products, such as soy beans and quinoa, are complete proteins, meaning that they contain all those essential amino acids that humans need. Others are missing some of these amino acids, so it is important to eat a varied diet. Amino acids are the building blocks of protein. Here are the top plant-based options for generating more protein in your diet that are easy to add to any meal:

- **Beans:** Beans contain more protein than any other vegetable protein and are packed with fibre, so you feel fuller for longer. Beans are an incomplete source of protein but add them to wholegrain rice and you have an easy five-minute dinner along with a complete protein meal that is low in fat and high in fibre, protein and carbs.

- **Nuts:** One serving of almonds gives you six grams of protein – nearly as much protein as one ounce of ribeye steak! You would need to eat a lot of almonds to match a full steak in terms of having a filling meal, but try adding a tablespoon of nut butter to your morning oats for a protein hit.

- **Seeds:** Seeds are low-calorie foods that are rich in fibre and heart-healthy omega-3 fatty acids. Chia seeds are a complete source of protein that contain two grams of protein per tablespoon. Similar to chia seeds, hemp seeds are a complete protein. Hemp seeds offer five grams of protein per tablespoon.

- **Whole grains:** An average slice of wholewheat bread gives you at least three grams of protein, along with fibre, again keeping you full for longer. Try pairing toast and peanut butter to make a complete plant-based protein snack.

- **Soy:** Soy products are among the richest sources of protein in a plant-based diet. Soy products also contain good levels of calcium and iron, which makes them healthful substitutes for dairy products.

- **Lentils and legumes:** Lentils contain a high amount of protein, fibre and key nutrients, including iron and potassium.

WHY DO WE NEED PROTEIN?

Macros aka macronutrients – carbs, fat and protein – play an important role in a balanced diet. Without going into too much detail (I would like to provide you with fun and useful information for daily health and wellness not a dissertation on how to become an advanced athlete!), carbohydrates are the body's main energy source, fat is important for you to be able to absorb vitamins A, D, E and K, and protein is important for building and repairing the body – which is why it is so important when you work out regularly. Weight training and other sports that put strain on your muscles need to be supported by a protein-rich yet well-balanced diet to ensure adequate muscle growth and recovery.

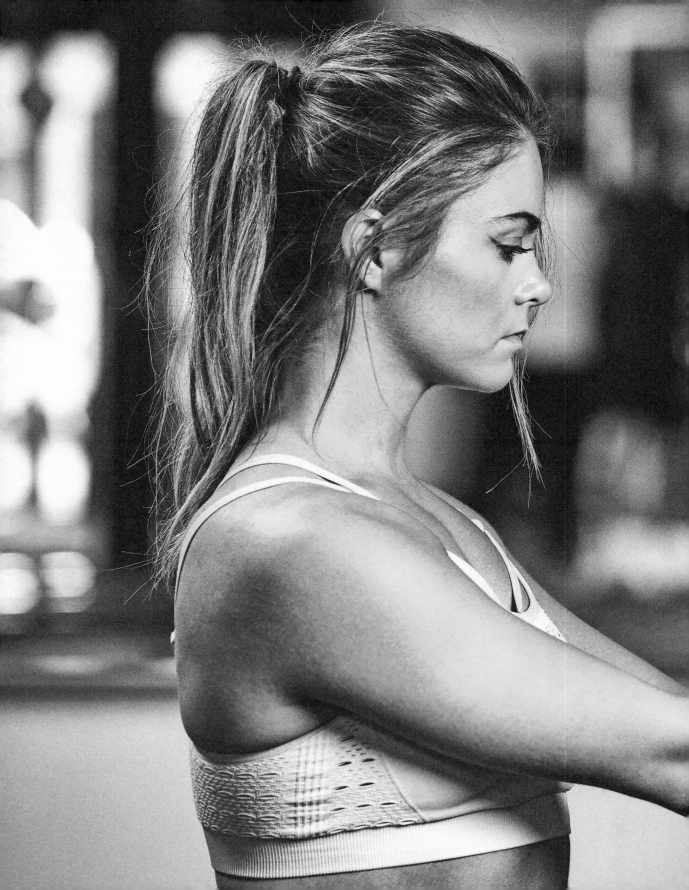

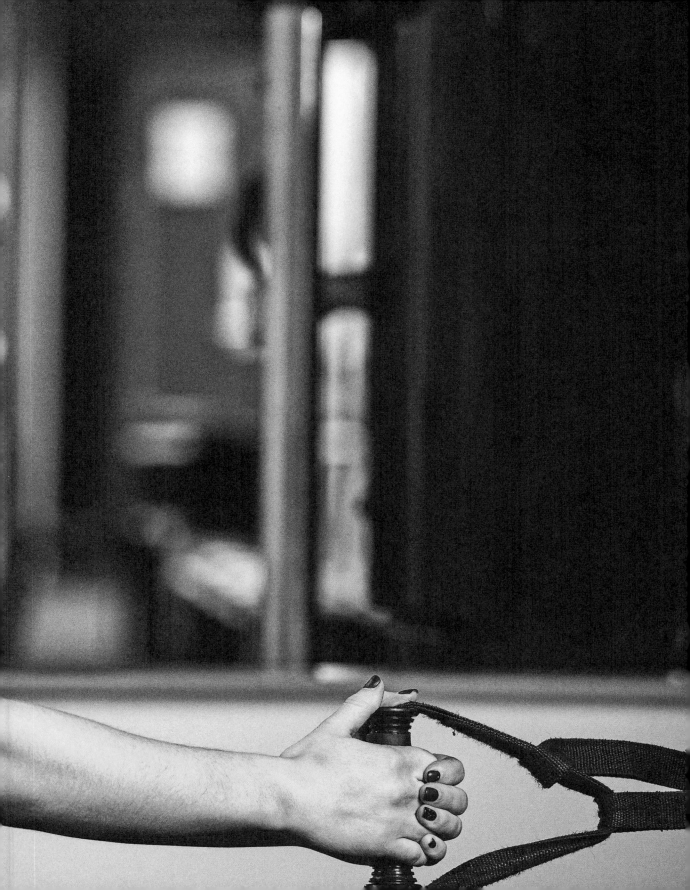

Protein is an important component of all cells in the body and is used for the growth and repair of tissues. I know that a lot of people immediately think of two things when protein is mentioned: bodybuilders and meat. But protein is not only important for gym-goers, nor – as I've shown – is it only found in animal products. Protein is essential for everyone – for strong hair, skin and nails, building and repairing muscle and to make enzymes, hormones and other body chemicals.

However, we need less protein than we might think. For example, I often get asked by 21-year-old girls, weighing 50kg, how they can hit 200g of protein on a plant-based diet. The human body does not typically need that much protein. Anyone who eats an eight-ounce steak typically served in restaurants is consuming more protein than their bodies can use. However, it is helpful to be aware of how much protein you are roughly getting – especially if you do have specific aesthetic goals in the gym.

The recipes in this book have a focus on protein and are designed to be 'macro-friendly'. That is, they are balanced and will fit in with your health and fitness goals, whether that be weight loss or muscle building, speed or agility. For example, rather than simply offering you up a recipe for a basic fruit smoothie, I add in protein sources to really bulk up the drink and make it an easy go-to breakfast or snack that will keep you feeling fuller and more satisfied for longer.

VITAMINS & SUPPLEMENTS

The main vitamins and minerals to be aware of on a plant-based diet are calcium, B12, iron, vitamin D and omega-3s. These are widely available in plant-based foods, so long as you make healthy choices. If you live a vegan lifestyle on non-dairy Ben & Jerry's and frozen pizza, then you might not get to where you want to be.

I personally find I receive enough nutrients if I make sure to incorporate the following foods in my diet:

- **Calcium:** rich leafy greens, beans and pulses, tofu and soy foods, dried fruit, sesame, flax and chia seeds.

- **Iron:** lentils, cannellini beans, soybeans, fortified oats, dark chocolate, chickpeas, tofu, tempeh, nuts, seeds and quinoa.

- **Omega-3:** chia seeds, walnuts, flaxseeds, seaweed, edamame beans.

As well as eating a balanced, nutrient-rich diet, I take a B12 and vitamin D supplement. Again, if you have any concerns or need further advice on what supplements you might take to suit your body, I would recommend seeking further advice before choosing the right path for you.

FREQUENTLY ASKED QUESTIONS

These are some of the questions I'm asked nearly every day. I hope that by addressing them here, I'll show you how veganism is possible for everyone and that it can make a real, positive difference both to your own wellbeing and to the planet.

WHAT ABOUT PROTEIN IN A VEGAN DIET?

People often ask this in relation to nutrition or training, without quite knowing what protein does and how much we actually need. I've found that it's not difficult to meet your protein requirements as a vegan and there are plenty of quality food sources to choose from.

If people are still unsure about my health, my response is to ask (with a smile!): 'Do I look undernourished? Do I look like there's not enough protein in my diet?'

BUT WHAT ABOUT COWS . . .

Dairy farming is centuries old, but factory farming, and farming on the huge scale that exists now, obviously isn't – and this is where the problem lies. Whether you are concerned for animal welfare or climate change, the demand for beef and cheap dairy products is taking its toll on the environment and on the wellbeing of the cows themselves. There are plenty of readily available plant-based sources of calcium to choose from instead – an optional, more ethical approach.

HOW WILL ONE PERSON GOING VEGAN MAKE A DIFFERENCE?

In an average lifetime, a meat eater in the Western world might well eat more than 7,000 animals. By choosing to reduce your meat consumption, animal suffering is reduced and the world's resources are saved. In its simplest terms, the rule of supply and demand means that when demand decreases sufficiently, so does supply. As more people buy fewer animal products, supermarket chains will gradually reduce their orders, and so fewer animals will be bred and killed, and fewer resources used.

The key is reduction – if you can cut your meat and dairy consumption down to once or twice a week rather than once or twice a day, you're hugely decreasing your impact on the planet and on animals.

BUT ISN'T VEGANISM EXPENSIVE?

Most of your cupboard essentials – like pasta, rice, beans, tinned tomatoes, lentils and fresh seasonal or frozen veggies – are relatively cheap, and you're likely to be buying those anyway whether or not you're eating a plant-based diet. Granted, meat alternatives can be expensive but if you compare the price of tofu to responsibly sourced meat, you will notice that in most cases the tofu will be cheaper.

ISN'T VEGANISM TOO EXTREME?
Livestock farming contributes more to climate change than all the cars, planes, ships and trains on the planet combined. It is also a significant factor in deforestation. A plant-based diet is kinder to the earth and all its animals, including the human race, while also having lots of health benefits. Unless you consider pasta, beans, peanut butter and bread to be extreme . . . there is nothing really extreme about not eating animals.

Instead of asking: '*Why don't you eat meat?*' perhaps the question should now be: '*Why do you eat meat?*'

VEGANISM IS SO RESTRICTIVE! I CAN'T EAT MY FAVOURITE FOODS!
When people tell me they can't go vegan because they'll miss meat or cheese too much, I usually say:

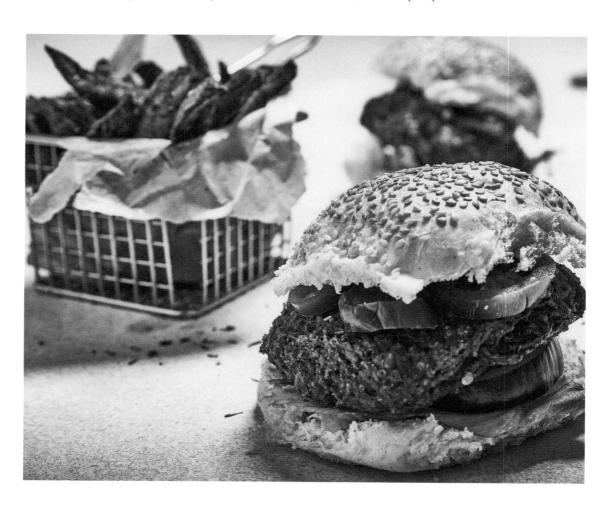

- You haven't got to go 'cold-turkey' and become a vegan overnight. You can take your time, gradually add more plants into your meals and slowly get used to living animal-product free. Think of it as eating in abundance, you're *adding* food to your diet rather than taking it away.

- You haven't got to be vegan. There, I said it! I'd be so happy if what you take away from this book is the inspiration to *reduce* your animal product intake, to really begin to love plants and yourself more. Small changes are just as important, and in making them you are still reducing your consumption and living a healthier lifestyle.

- Many of your favourite food items may already be vegan! I once created a popular series on my YouTube channel where I hunted down my favourite 'accidentally vegan' junk foods and showcased them in videos to demonstrate how much of your everyday favourites might already be animal-free!

- With the vegan movement growing more and more each day there are now alternatives to just about everything. My supermarket freezer section is exploding with dairy-free pizza, meat-free sausages and burgers. I don't know what restrictive means to you, but this sure isn't it.

BUT WILL VEGANISM MAKE ME FEEL BETTER?

For many of us, our relationship to food is complicated. Deciding to no longer eat certain foods that you love, that bring you comfort or that your body has come to rely on is hard.

However, as you transition to a more plant-based diet, the benefits of eating this way will eventually start to balance out the sadness you feel at no longer eating a meaty cheeseburger . . . trust me, I've never felt better! And, surprise, you can still enjoy vegan cheeseburgers!

WARM-UP

It's my passion to help you live a healthier, happier and stronger life through good food, exercise and daily routines. It isn't rocket science and there's no magic pill, just a few small changes to your everyday life, so you hopefully take from the pages of *Naturally Stefanie* a fresh new energy for your life.

Remember: 'Be happy, life is once.'

Stefanie x

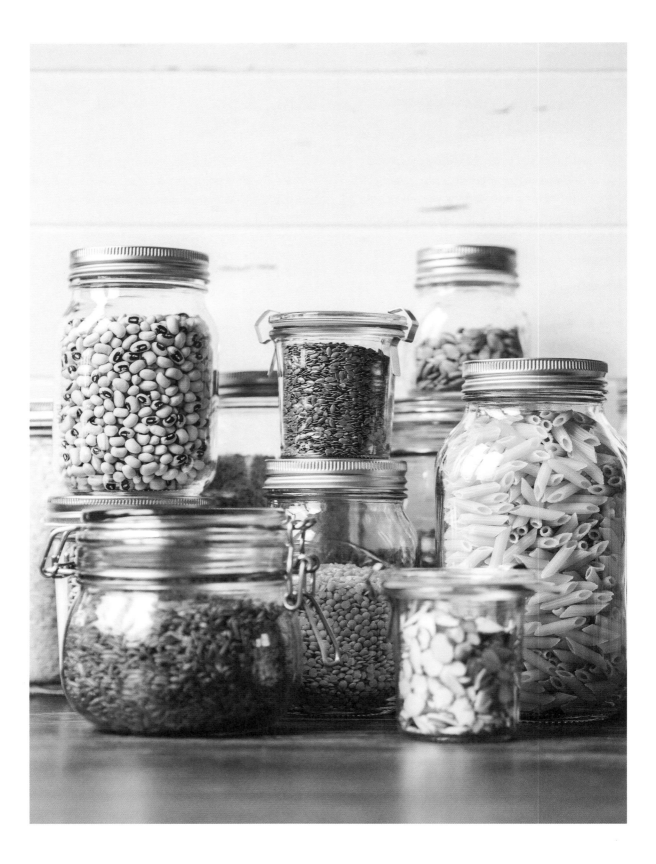

KITCHEN STAPLES

These are some of the everyday foods that my recipes use. With a well-stocked kitchen, you can always make yourself a healthy, easy meal.

RICE
I use different rice types depending on the dish; jasmine, pilau, wholegrain and basmati are some of my favourites.

PASTA
I have found that supermarkets now have every kind of pasta you can imagine – high protein pasta, lentil pasta, pasta made from chickpeas, gluten free and so on. I use a mixture of wholewheat penne and lentil pasta.

NOODLES
The noodles in this book can be replaced with whatever variety you prefer. However, I always use either wholewheat or rice noodles in my recipes.

TOFU
For the main meal recipes, make sure you use firm tofu (and make sure it's drained of moisture before cooking). For puddings and desserts, I use silken tofu, which has a different consistency.

TEMPEH
Tempeh is not quite as easy to get your hands on as meat alternatives such as tofu, for example. It can usually be sourced in health food stores, specialised supermarkets or online. It is similar to tofu in that it is a protein source but it has a much firmer and almost nuttier texture to it.

SEITAN
Like tempeh, you can find seitan in health foods stores and online. It is also a great protein source, providing a meaty texture to dishes.

NUT AND SEED BUTTERS
Nut butters are a great way of adding protein and flavour to meals but, again, if you can't eat nuts, switching nuts, switching up any nut butters with seed butters is a great alternative. For example, sunflower seed butter is a fabulous replacement for peanut butter.

BEANS AND LENTILS
There are a variety of different beans and lentils you can use throughout the recipes. I always recommend having tinned black beans, chickpeas, white beans and kidney beans at hand, and a selection of both tinned and dried lentils.

OATS
Nothing fancy needed here – basic rolled oats are all you need for a brilliant bowl of heart-warming porridge or to blend into fluffy pancakes.

PROTEIN POWDER

I have included this in a few of the breakfast recipes to add a protein punch to basic smoothies. However, it is optional and you can omit if you do not have it to hand. Similarly, in the cooked recipes such as pancakes or waffles merely substitute the same amount of flour for protein powder. Using the protein powder will *not* make you bulky; it provides the protein source for a meal in the same way that beans, for example, would to your dinner.

PLANT-BASED MILK

I personally love using almond milk (particularly in my smoothies), but if you can't eat nuts, I recommend using a plant-based milk of your choice, such as coconut milk or oat milk, instead.

VEGAN CHEESE

Vegan cheese – in many forms! – can now be found in most supermarkets and health food stores. Some of the recipes require mozzarella-like cheese, so I recommend you try a few options until you find a variety that suits you.

SPICES AND SEASONING

A combination of dried and fresh herbs and spices are required throughout this book. Once you have stocked up your spice cupboard, you will find you have more than enough to last you months!

FRUIT AND VEGETABLES

Fresh fruits and vegetables are optimal for a healthy diet. But, of course, having some frozen berries and vegetables in your freezer is also a great, super convenient way to stay on track. Throw frozen veggies into your meals or berries into your smoothies to be an easy step closer to your five-a-day.

DAIRY-FREE CHOCOLATE

It goes without saying that chocolate is a staple item in my kitchen. Anything dairy-free works in these recipes and, just as with the vegan cheese, I suggest you give a range of different dairy-free chocolate a try, so you can find one that really works for you.

KITCHEN EQUIPMENT

Nothing fancy required, but a food processer and a blender are vital for a lot of the recipes in this book. A juicer and a waffle maker aren't as essential but will be needed if you're interested in making juices and waffles! Apart from that, your basic kitchen equipment – a couple of sharp knives, non-stick pans, tubs for food storage, a grater and a garlic mincer – will be all you need to get cooking.

BLENDER

I personally use a Vitamix – which is quite the fancy blender. However, as long as your blender can break up frozen fruit and ice, you are good to go!

FOOD PROCESSOR

This is so useful for making recipes such as protein balls and you'll soon find that a good food processor is a really worthwhile addition to your kitchen.

JUICER

Again, you do not need anything fancy here, but it is worth noting that this kitchen kit is used nearly every day, so it makes sense to invest in something reasonably good quality, but not too pricey, so you won't need to replace it every month.

WAFFLE MAKER

Top tip – buy a non-stick waffle maker online for less than £30. Key words being *non-stick*!

NON-STICK PANS

These are handy if, like me, you don't use a lot of oil. They also last longer as you don't need to scrub them when washing off food that has got burned on to them.

GRATER

A standard box grater does the job just fine!

GARLIC MINCER OR PRESS

This handy tool will save you lots of time when prepping ingredients.

KITCHEN KNIVES

Again, nothing fancy, just a standard bread knife and chopping knife, but keep them nice and sharp.

TUBS AND STORAGE FOR MEAL PREP OR LEFTOVERS

These are optional, but they are great to store any leftover food for your lunch the next day or for meal prepping.

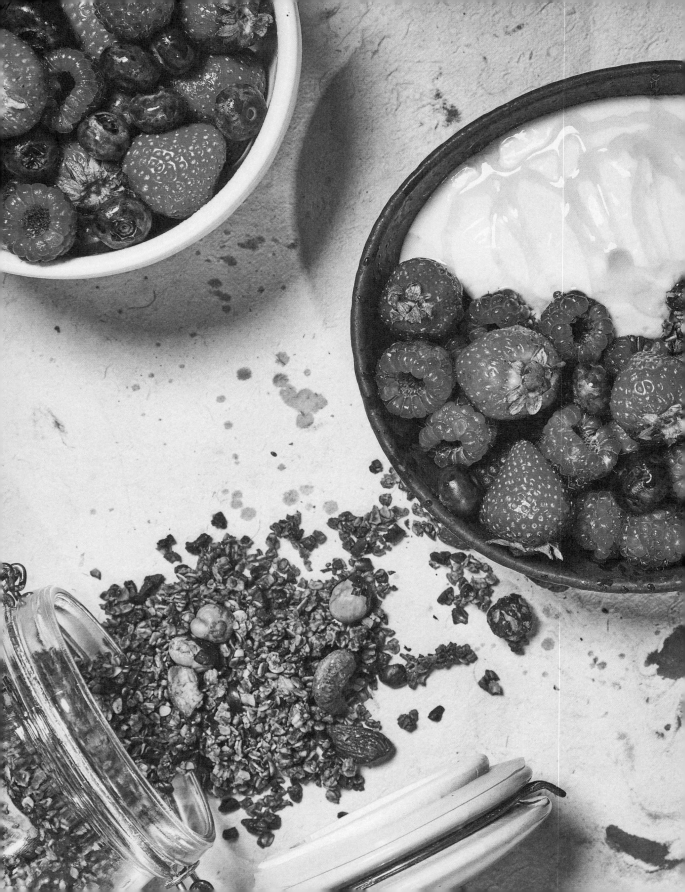

BREAKFASTS

SMOOTHIES

Chocolate lovers	20
Chocolate maca	20
Peanut butter oatmeal	20
No protein powder	20
Ultimate recovery	20
Mango and ginger	22
Acai black forest	22
Green goddess	22

JUICES

Post workout hulk	25
Immunity boost	25
Ginger shot	25
Antioxidant punch	25
Beat it	25
Watermelon lime cooler	25
Protein-packed iced coffee	25

PANCAKES – 5 WAYS

Banana with chocolate sauce	26
Chocolate chip	27
Caramelised banana and pecan	27
Strawberries and cream	28
Blueberry and lemon	28

BREAKFASTS

PORRIDGE – 3 WAYS

WAFFLES – 2 WAYS

BREAKFASTS

SMOOTHIES

Each recipe makes 1 smoothie

For all of these smoothies, simply blend all of the ingredients together in a blender or food processor until smooth. For all of the smoothies, both fresh and frozen ingredients work well. I often like using frozen fruit and veg, so my smoothies are nice and cold – and refreshing.

CHOCOLATE LOVERS

2 bananas
2 tbsp raw cacao powder
2 tbsp oats
40g vegan chocolate protein powder, optional
1 tbsp almond butter (or seed butter)
230ml almond milk

CHOCOLATE MACA

2 bananas
2 tbsp raw cacao powder
40g vegan chocolate protein powder, optional
1 tsp maca powder
1 tsp lucuma powder
230ml almond milk

PEANUT BUTTER OATMEAL

2 bananas
2 tbsp oats
1 tbsp peanut butter (or sunflower seed butter)
40g vegan vanilla protein powder, optional
230ml almond milk
60g soy yogurt

NO PROTEIN POWDER

This smoothie delivers an amazing 19g of protein without using any protein powder!

100g fresh spinach
2 bananas
150g frozen mango
230ml coconut water
1 tbsp chia seeds
1 tbsp flax seeds
1 tbsp almond butter (or seed butter)

ULTIMATE RECOVERY

Combining carbohydrates, proteins, and some fats after exercising helps to encourage muscle protein production and recovery.

2 bananas
150g berries
230ml coconut water
40g vegan vanilla protein powder, optional
1 tsp turmeric

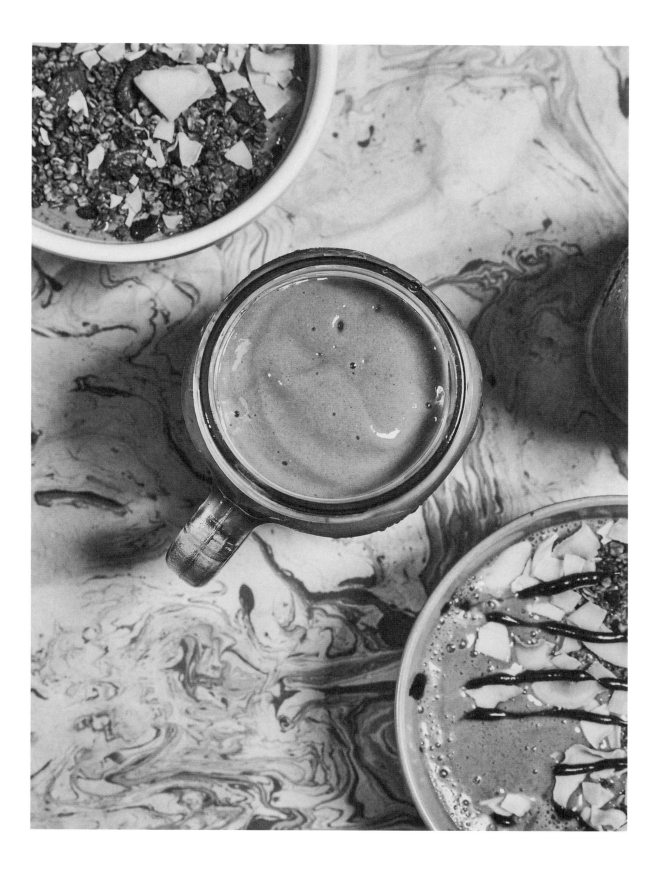

MANGO AND GINGER

Research has shown that ginger helps reduce inflammation post-workout and can assist in speeding up muscle recovery. Taking as little as 1.5 teaspoons of fresh ginger daily can reduce delayed onset muscle soreness (DOMS) up to 25 per cent.

300g frozen mango
230ml almond milk
120g vegan soy yogurt
1 tsp fresh ginger, grated
1 tsp turmeric

ACAI BLACK FOREST

1 frozen banana
150g frozen berries
40g vanilla protein powder, optional
230ml almond milk
1 tbsp acai powder

GREEN GODDESS

Spinach contains iron for energy and can also help improve endurance. Other benefits of spinach include helping to boost immunity and improving bone and skin health.

1-2 handfuls of spinach
1-2 handfuls of kale
230ml almond milk
150g pineapple, fresh or tinned
150g frozen mango
½ apple, cored with the skin left on
½ lime, juiced

SMOOTHIE BOWLS

Any of the smoothies in this book can be turned into smoothie bowls by simply pouring the smoothie into a bowl and adding some delicious toppings, such as fresh berries, coconut flakes, chia seeds, homemade granola and cacao nibs.

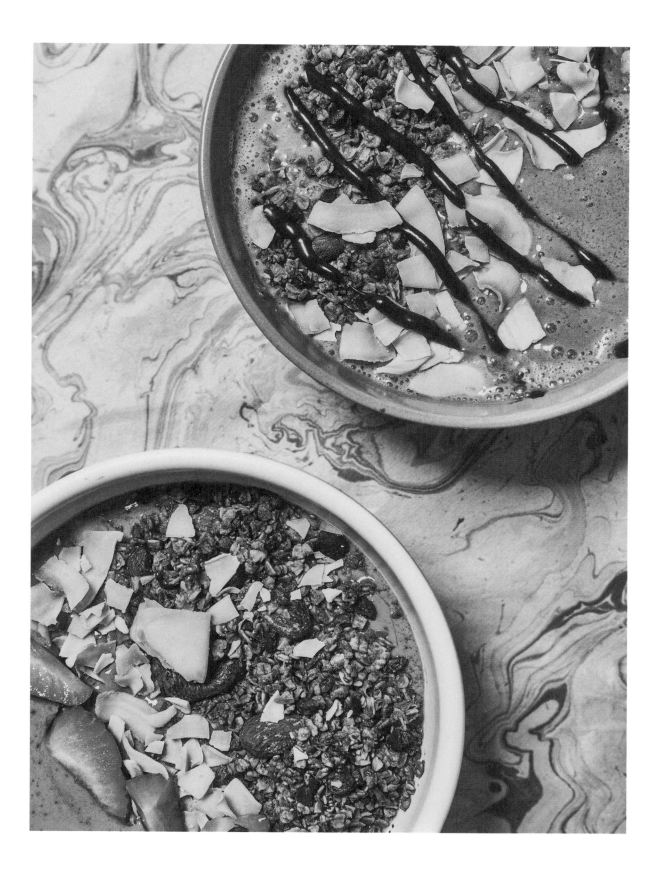

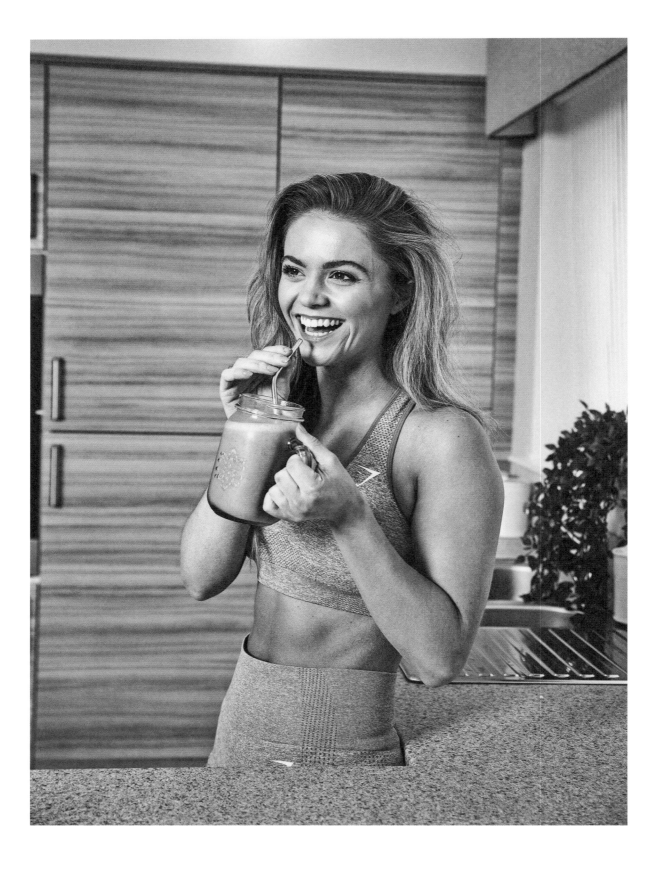

JUICES

Each recipe makes 1 large juice

For all of the juices, simply wash and then run all of the ingredients through a juicer and mix well, then add ice. I like to use fresh ingredients in these juices but tinned and frozen are also delicious. Make sure you let any frozen produce thaw before juicing!

POST WORKOUT HULK

2 apples, cored and sliced
1 celery stalk
1 lime, peeled and cut into quarters
1-2 handfuls of spinach
1-2 handfuls of kale
½ cucumber (leave the skin on if it's organic!)

IMMUNITY BOOST

2 carrots, leave unpeeled if organic
1 apple, cored and sliced
1 orange, peeled and cut into quarters
½ lemon, peeled and halved

GINGER SHOT

¼ pineapple
2-inch piece of ginger root, grated

ANTIOXIDANT PUNCH

10 strawberries
2 fresh beetroots, washed and peeled
300g blueberries

BEAT IT

1 fresh beetroot, washed and peeled
1 apple, cored and sliced
1 celery stalk
¼ pineapple, fresh or tinned
¼ cucumber (leave the skin on if it's organic!)

WATERMELON LIME COOLER

8 strawberries
2 limes, peeled and cut into quarters
½ watermelon

PROTEIN-PACKED ICED COFFEE

This incredible drink will really set you up pre-workout!

2 tbsp raw cacao powder
100g ice
230ml almond milk
1 tbsp maple syrup
1 tsp vanilla extract
½ tbsp coffee (instant or ground are equally good)

PANCAKES – 5 WAYS

Each recipe makes 6–8 pancakes

I often make these recipes for family and friends. If you're cooking a large batch of pancakes, I would recommend keeping the cooked pancakes warm in the oven on a low heat, so everyone can eat together.

The trick with all these pancakes is to make sure the centre of the pancake is cooked through – not just the outside. My poor husband, Marco, has been subject to a few too many soggy pancakes in his time!

Leave your pancake mix to sit for ten minutes before cooking so it thickens up and is not runny. Then cook on a low to medium heat and allow the pancakes to cook slowly until the edges start browning and little holes or bubbles appear in the batter – that's when you know the centre is cooking. No soggy pancakes here – hooray!

1. BANANA WITH CHOCOLATE SAUCE

Ingredients

200ml almond milk
100g oats
35g vegan vanilla protein powder or
    substitute with 35g of oats
1 ripe banana
1 tsp baking powder
1 banana, chopped, for topping

For the chocolate sauce

1 tbsp maple syrup
1 tsp raw cacao powder

1. Lightly grease and preheat a non-stick frying pan over a medium heat.

2. Using a blender or whisk, mix together the pancake ingredients to form a smooth batter.

3. Once the pan is hot, pour the batter into the pan until desired pancake size is reached.

4. Cook the pancakes until the surface begins to bubble and the edges turn brown then flip and cook on the other side. This should take between 4 and 6 minutes.

5. Remove from the heat and transfer to your plate or into the oven to stay warm.

6. For the chocolate sauce, mix together the maple syrup and cacao powder and pour liberally over your pancakes, adding the chopped banana as a finishing touch. Enjoy!

BREAKFASTS

2. CHOCOLATE CHIP

Ingredients

200ml almond milk
100g oats
35g vegan chocolate protein powder or
    substitute with 25g of oats and
    2 tbsp cacao powder
2 tbsp vegan-friendly chocolate chips
1 ripe banana
1 tsp baking powder

Toppings

1 tbsp maple syrup
handful of vegan-friendly chocolate chips

1. Lightly grease and preheat non-stick frying pan over a medium heat.

2. Using a blender or whisk, combine the pancake ingredients to form a smooth batter. Once blended, stir in the chocolate chips.

3. Once the pan is hot, pour the batter into the pan until desired pancake size is reached.

4. Cook the pancakes until the surface begins to bubble and the edges turn brown then flip and cook on the other side. This should take between 4 and 6 minutes.

5. Remove from the heat and transfer to your plate or into the oven to stay warm.

6. Top with chocolate chips and maple syrup.

3. CARAMELISED BANANA AND PECAN

Ingredients

200ml almond milk
100g oats
35g vegan vanilla protein powder or
    substitute with 35g of oats
1 tbsp pecans
1 ripe banana
1 tsp baking powder

Toppings

1 banana
1 tbsp pecans
1 tbsp coconut sugar

1. Lightly grease and preheat a non-stick frying pan over a medium heat.

2. Using a blender or whisk, combine the pancake ingredients to form a smooth batter. Once blended, crush 1 tbsp of pecans and stir into the mixture.

3. Pour the batter into the pre-heated pan until desired pancake size is reached.

4. Cook the pancakes until the surface begins to bubble and the edges turn brown then flip and cook on the other side. This should take between 4 and 6 minutes. Remove from heat and transfer to your plate or into the oven to stay warm.

5. As your pancakes are cooking, add the banana and your tbsp of the whole pecans to a baking tray.

6. Lightly dust the banana and pecans with the coconut sugar and place under the grill until golden. Remove from the heat and add to your stack of pancakes.

4. STRAWBERRIES AND CREAM

Ingredients

200ml almond milk
100g oats
35g vegan vanilla protein powder or
   substitute with 35g of oats
1 ripe banana
1 tsp baking powder

Toppings

150g strawberries, chopped
2 tbsp soya cream
1 tbsp maple syrup

1. Lightly grease and preheat a non-stick frying pan over a medium heat.

2. Using a blender or whisk, combine the pancake ingredients to form a smooth batter.

3. Once the pan is hot, pour the batter into the pan until desired pancake size is reached.

4. Cook the pancakes until the surface begins to bubble and the edges turn brown then flip and cook on the other side. This should take between 4 and 6 minutes.

5. Remove from the heat and transfer to your plate or into the oven to stay warm.

6. Top with chopped strawberries, soya cream and maple syrup.

5. BLUEBERRY AND LEMON

Ingredients

200ml almond milk
100g oats
35g vegan vanilla protein powder or
   substitute with 35g of oats
1 ripe banana
1 tsp baking powder
150g blueberries (plus extra for topping)
juice and zest of 1 lemon

1. First, juice and zest the lemon. Set the zest to one side – you'll use it as a topping for the pancakes later

2. Lightly grease and preheat a non-stick pan over a medium heat.

3. Using a blender or whisk, mix together the oats, protein powder, banana, baking powder, lemon juice and almond milk to form a smooth batter. Then add the blueberries.

4. Once the pan is hot, pour the batter into the pan until desired pancake size is reached.

5. Cook the pancakes until the surface begins to bubble and the edges turn brown then flip and cook on the other side. This should take between 4 and 6 minutes.

6. Remove from the heat and transfer to your plate or into the oven to stay warm.

7. Top with the extra blueberries and lemon zest.

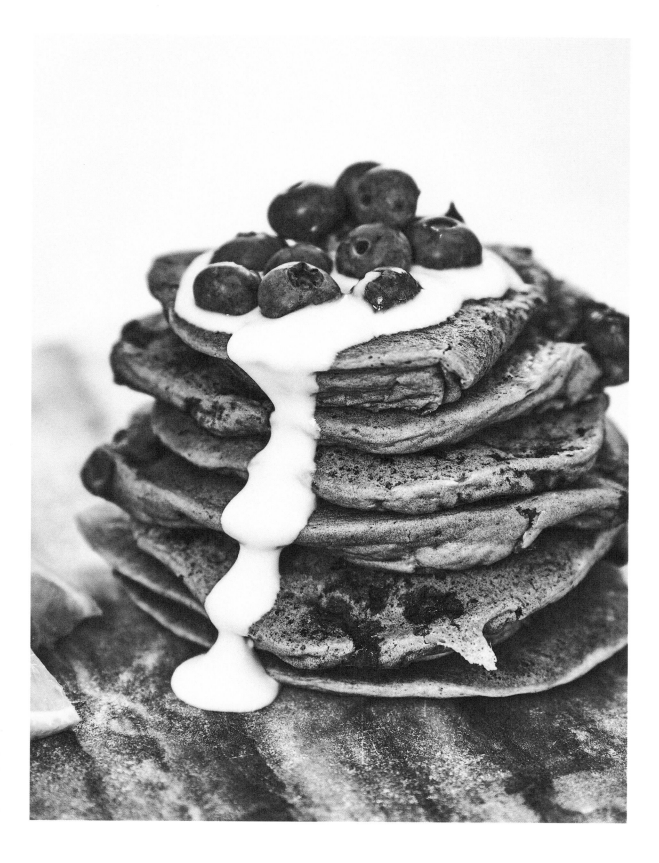

PORRIDGE – 3 WAYS

Each recipe makes 1 bowl of porridge

Oats are a great source of carbohydrates and fibre and are also higher in protein and fat than most other grains. They are also very high in many vitamins and minerals such as folate, manganese, magnesium, copper, iron and zinc. Their carbohydrate content makes them incredibly beneficial for preparing your muscles for working out. They are also digested at a slow pace which means that eating them as a pre-workout meal will result in intra-workout energising benefits. Porridge is a filling and warming breakfast that will keep you sustained into the afternoon.

1. ALMOND BUTTER AND JAM

Ingredients

100-150ml almond milk or a plant-based
   milk of your choice
50g porridge oats
1 tsp cinnamon

Toppings

1 tbsp chia seeds jam (page 129)
1 tbsp creamy almond butter
1 tbsp maple syrup

1. Add the oats, almond milk and cinnamon to a saucepan and cook over a high heat.

2. Bring the mixture to a boil, then turn down the heat, leaving the porridge to simmer until you reach your desired consistency – depending on how soft you like your oats. Alternatively, use a microwave to do this – I would recommend a cooking time of 5 minutes.

3. Once the desired consistency has been reached, remove the porridge from the heat and transfer into a bowl.

4. Top with runny almond butter, jam and maple syrup.

2. CHOCOLATE AND PEANUT BUTTER

Ingredients

100-150ml almond milk
50g porridge oats
2 tbsp raw cacao powder
2 tbsp maple syrup

Toppings

1 tbsp peanut butter
1 tbsp raw cacao nibs
1 tbsp toasted coconut flakes

1. Add the oats, almond milk, cacao powder and 1 tbsp of maple syrup into a saucepan over a high heat.

2. Bring the mixture to a boil, then turn down the heat, leaving the porridge to simmer until you reach your desired consistency – depending on how soft you like your oats. Alternatively, use a microwave to do this – I would recommend a cooking time of 5 minutes.

3. Once the desired consistency has been reached, remove the porridge from the heat and transfer to a bowl.

4. Top with the peanut butter, cacao nibs, coconut flakes and the remaining maple syrup.

OVERNIGHT OATS

You can take any of these porridge recipes and make them into overnight oats – a great solution to a healthy breakfast if you are short on time in the morning. Simply mix all of the ingredients for each recipe into a Mason jar or tub and store in the fridge overnight to grab and go the next day. No cooking required as the oats 'cook' overnight and the porridge can be eaten cold!

3. GRILLED PEAR AND COCONUT

Ingredients

100-150ml coconut milk
50g porridge oats
1 tsp cinnamon
1 tbsp desiccated coconut

Toppings

1-2 grilled pears, sliced
1 tbsp maple syrup

For the grilled pears

2 pears
½ tsp of olive oil

For the grilled pears

1. Halve the pears, remove the cores and brush with a little olive oil.

2. Heat a grill pan over a medium heat and place the pears, face down, on the grill.

3. Cook for around 10 minutes until the pears begin to soften.

For the porridge

1. Add the oats, coconut milk, desiccated coconut and cinnamon into saucepan over a high heat.

2. Bring the mixture to a boil, then turn down the heat, leaving the porridge to simmer until you reach your desired consistency – depending on how soft you like your oats. Alternatively, you can use a microwave to do this – I would recommend a cooking time of 5 minutes.

3. Once the desired consistency has been reached, remove the porridge from the heat and transfer to a bowl.

4. Top with the grilled pear if you prefer, (you can always use fresh pears) and maple syrup.

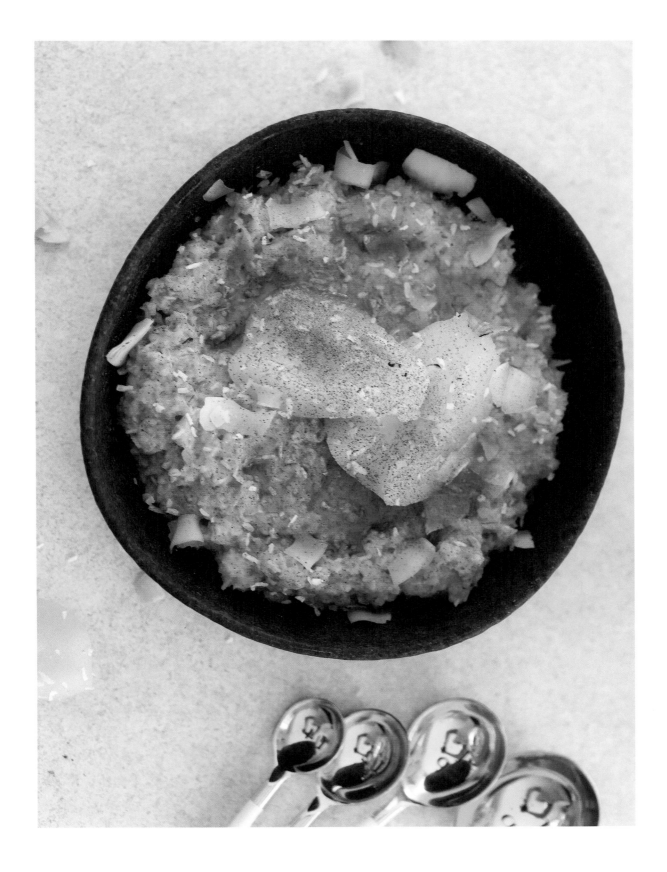

WAFFLES – 2 WAYS

Each recipe makes 2 waffles

A word of advice on waffles

Invest in a decent non-stick waffle maker, and by 'invest' I mean spend no more than £30. Trust me, do not buy a waffle maker that is not non-stick because your waffle will look like it has been through a few wars by the time you are done with it.

My first attempt at making waffles (yes, here I go again!) was somewhat tragic. Imagine my excitement at the delivery man dropping off my newly purchased waffle maker. I walked briskly (okay, I ran) to my kitchen and set it up before whipping up a basic waffle batter to test it out. This is where it went drastically wrong. The batter was fine, there was nothing wrong with the actual recipe itself. It was the waffle maker that was the problem.

Imagine opening the waffle maker like a kid unwrapping a Christmas present only to find out your toy was broken, and you couldn't play with it – a little dramatic, but my waffle was the toy in this scenario. The waffle had stuck in lumps and clumps to the top and bottom of the machine, burned on the corners, was spilling out the sides – yet the middle was wet and mushy. Using a fork, I scraped together the 'waffle' and plopped it on the plate. Then I looked at this abomination in dismay.

Moral of the story: buy a good, non-stick waffle maker.

1. CHOCOLATE CHIP

Ingredients

120ml almond milk
70g oats
30g vegan vanilla protein powder or
    substitute with 30g of oats
2 tbsp vegan-friendly chocolate chips, plus
    extra for topping
1 tsp baking powder
1 banana

Toppings

1 banana, sliced
1 tbsp maple syrup
vegan-friendly chocolate chips

1. First, preheat the waffle maker.

2. While it heats up, mix the oats, protein powder, baking powder, banana and almond milk in a blender – the mixture should be much thicker than pancake batter.

3. If you're making the chocolate chip waffles, add the chocolate chips to the finished batter.

4. Add the batter to the waffle maker and cook for 5 minutes.

5. Remove the waffle once cooked. It should be golden brown and slightly crispy.

6. Top with either the sliced banana, maple syrup and extra chocolate chips or the raspberries.

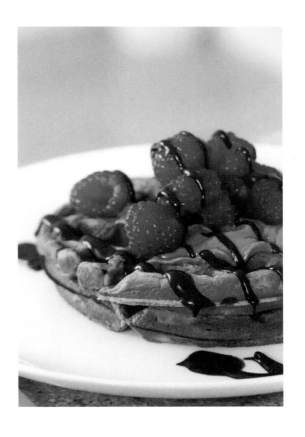

2. VANILLA AND RASPBERRY

Ingredients

120ml almond milk
70g oats
30g vegan vanilla protein powder or
    substitute with 30g of oats
1 tsp baking powder
1 ripe banana

Toppings

150g raspberries

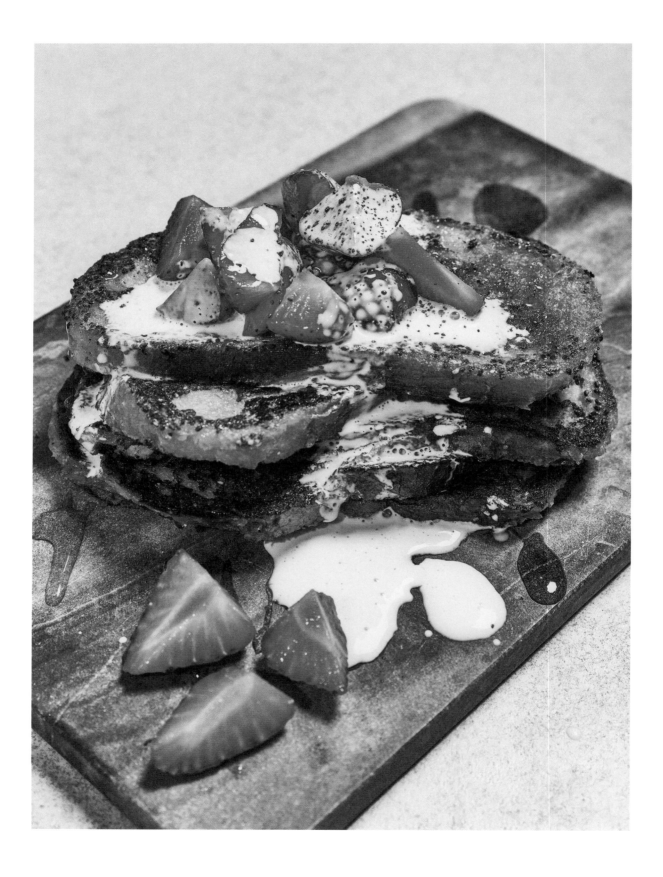

CHIA SEED FRENCH TOAST

Serves 2

Perfect for a lazy weekend brunch, this recipe is a vegan twist on an old favourite.
Chia seeds and soya cream add an extra punch of plant protein!

Ingredients

4 slices of bread, of your choice
230ml almond milk
1 tbsp maple syrup
1 tbsp chia seeds
¼ tsp vanilla
¼ tsp nutmeg
¼ tsp ginger

Toppings

2 tbsp soya cream
1 tbsp maple syrup
150g strawberries, chopped

1. In a bowl, whisk together the almond milk, maple syrup, spices, chia seeds, nutmeg, ginger and vanilla and let sit for 5 minutes.

2. Preheat a non-stick frying pan over a medium heat and lightly grease with some coconut oil.

3. Evenly coat one of the slices of bread into the chia seed mix and transfer it to the pan to cook until golden brown. Repeat with the other 3 slices of bread, or until the chia seed mixture is used up.

4. Remove the toast from the pan and top with the strawberries, soya cream and maple syrup.

TURMERIC TOFU SCRAMBLE

Serves 1

The vegan alter ego to scrambled eggs – great on toast or part of your Ultimate British Breakfast.

Ingredients

200g tofu
½ red onion, chopped
2 cloves garlic, minced
1 big bunch spinach, stems removed
1 tsp turmeric
1 tsp paprika
1 tsp black pepper
1 tsp salt
1 tbsp soy sauce
2 slices of wholemeal bread

1. Drain and pat dry your tofu to remove excess moisture.

2. Crumble your tofu into small chunks and cook in a non-stick pan over a medium heat for around 5 to 7 minutes or until starting to brown.

3. Add in the vegetables and cook for another 5 minutes until vegetables have softened.

4. Mix in the soy sauce and spices and coat the tofu and vegetables evenly.

5. Add scramble to freshly toasted bread.

SPRINKLE-ON-EVERYTHING GRANOLA

Makes 1 large jar

As the name suggests, this granola is an amazing addition to any sweet breakfast dish. I love it with yogurt and berries, but it also adds an extra crunch to smoothie bowls and is perfect as an additional topping on homemade pancakes.

Ingredients

240g oats
240g unsalted mixed nuts
2 tbsp raw cacao nibs
2 tbsp chia seeds
2 tbsp maple syrup
2 tbsp coconut oil
1 tsp vanilla extract

1. Preheat the oven to 140°C.

2. In a large mixing bowl, combine all the dry ingredients and set to one side.

3. Add the coconut oil to a small saucepan and cook it over a low heat until melted. Remove from heat and stir in the maple syrup and vanilla extract.

4. Add the wet mixture to the dry ingredients and mix together well.

5. Spread the granola on a baking tray and place in the oven for 45 minutes, stirring every 10 minutes to prevent burning.

6. Allow to cool then store in an airtight container. This should last a month or two.

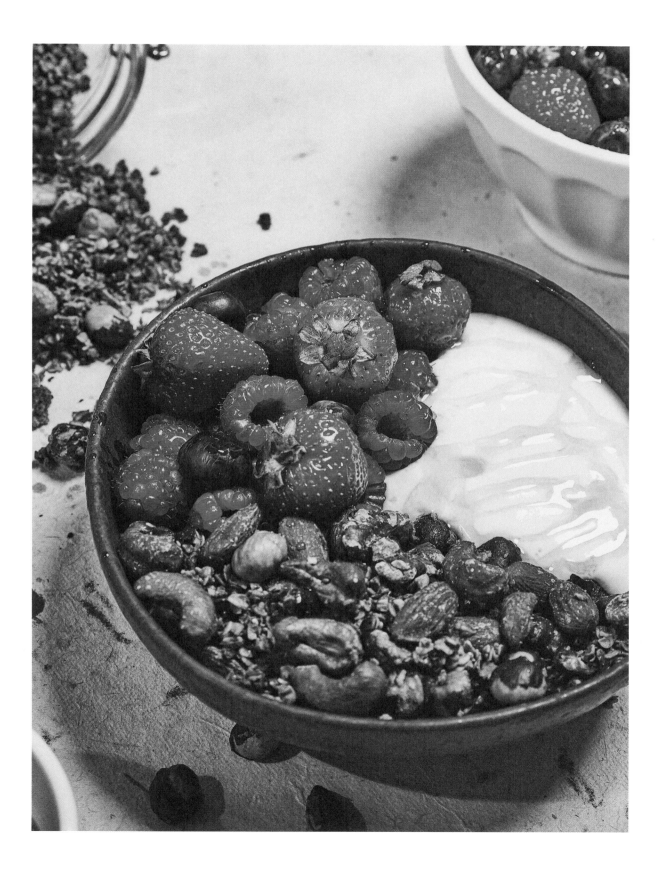

THE ULTIMATE BRITISH BREAKFAST

Makes 1 hearty portion

I think it is only fitting that this book contains the ultimate Sunday breakfast treat.
Behold the big British fry-up – with a healthy, vegan twist.

Ingredients

2 vegan-friendly
  sausages
2 slices wholemeal
  bread, to toast
1 large baking potato,
  cut into 1cm cubes

For the turmeric tofu
vegetable scramble

200g tofu, drained
100g mushrooms,
  chopped into chunks
100g cherry tomatoes,
  halved
½ red onion, finely
  chopped
1 big bunch spinach,
  stalks removed
1 tsp turmeric
1 tsp paprika
1 tsp black pepper
1 tsp salt
1 tbsp soy sauce

1. Preheat your oven to 180°C.

2. Cut the potato into 1cm cubes and steam or boil until cooked through – this should take around 15 minutes.

3. Once cooked, transfer the potato to a baking tray and roast the potatoes in the oven for a further 10 to 15 minutes.

4. For the sausages, check the cooking time as per the package instructions. I would recommend adding the sausages to the oven, so they are ready around the same time as the potatoes.

5. Now you can cook the tofu vegetable scramble once your sausages and potatoes are in the oven.

6. Grease and preheat a non-stick frying pan over a medium heat.

7. Chop the mushrooms, tomatoes and onion and crumble your tofu into small chunks.

8. Add the tofu to the pan. Cook for around 5 to 7 minutes or until the tofu starts to brown.

9. Add the mushrooms, tomatoes, onion and spinach to the pan and cook for another 5 minutes

10. In a separate bowl, mix the soy sauce and spices together, then add to the pan, coating the tofu and vegetables evenly.

11. Pop your bread in the toaster as you begin to assemble your breakfast.

12. Remove the tofu vegetable scramble from the heat and add to your plate, alongside the sausages, potatoes and toast. Serve with your favourite vegan breakfast sauce – happy Sunday!

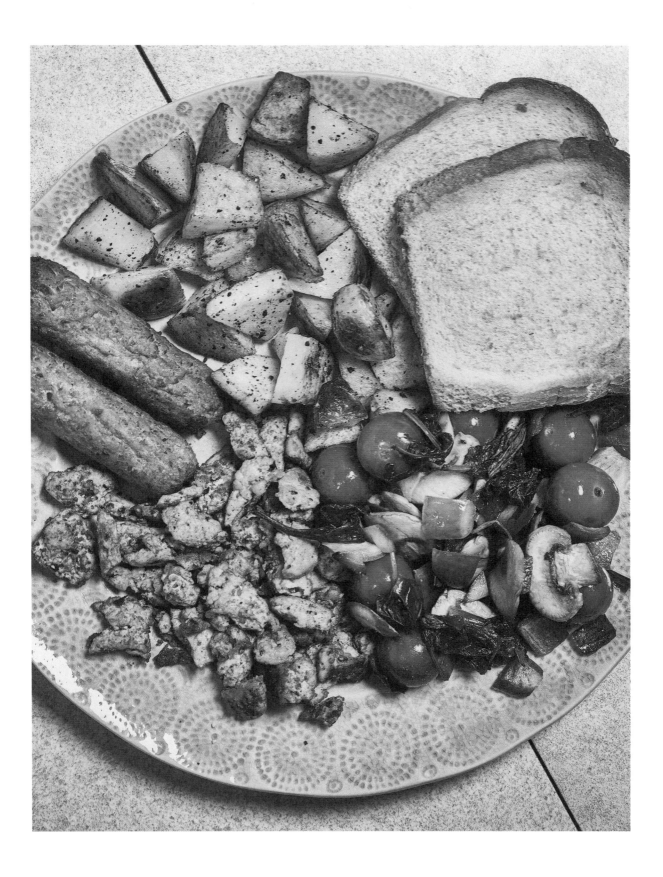

BREAKFAST – ALL WRAPPED UP

Serves 1

I love making wraps for breakfast – they're quick, easy and make for a hearty first meal of the day. Like my nourish bowls (page 55), you can simply add whatever sweet or savoury breakfast foods you have available and wrap them up in a tortilla of your choice – perfect for when you're heading out the door in the morning. I often add leftovers to my wraps so some of the food options below mention some of my favourite recipes that taste amazing all wrapped up!

1. WRAP: Choose one

- Plain tortilla
- Wholemeal tortilla
- Multiseed tortilla
- Corn tortilla
- Gluten-free tortilla
- Coconut tortilla
- Sweet potato tortilla

2. FRUIT & VEGETABLES: Choose three

- Spinach
- Pepper
- Onion
- Mushroom
- Potato
- Sweet potato
- Kale
- Tomato
- Fresh berries of your choice
- Banana
- Apple or pear
- Desiccated coconut

3. PROTEIN & FATS: Choose one

- Tofu scramble (page 38)
- Breakfast fritters (page 45)
- Sweet potato and tempeh hash (page 47)
- Haggis bon bons (page 125)
- Black beans
- Chilli beans
- Vegan-friendly sausages
- Avocado
- Flax seeds
- Hemp seeds
- Chia seeds
- Pumpkin seeds
- Sesame seeds
- Vegan cheese
- Nut butter
- Seed butter

4. DRESSING: Choose one

- Guacamole (page 126)
- Hummus (page 126)
- Salsa (page 127)
- Avocado and herb dressing (page 128)
- Easy peasy pesto (page 128)
- Chia strawberry jam (page 129)
- Chocolate fudge sauce (page 129)
- Vegan yogurt
- Maple syrup

BREAKFASTS

BLACK BEAN AND AVOCADO
BREAKFAST WRAP

Makes 2

*Perfect for any time of the day but especially good as a savoury breakfast option. I like
to double the recipe, so I have leftovers for breakfast or lunch the next day, too.*

Ingredients

2 wholemeal tortilla wraps
1 tin black beans, drained and rinsed
1 sweet potato, peeled
1 avocado, sliced
2 garlic cloves
½ white onion
handful of kale
2 tbsp hot sauce

1. Cut your sweet potato into small chunks and either steam or boil until cooked through – this should take around 15 minutes.

2. Finely chop the onion and garlic and add to a preheated frying pan with the kale. Cook for a few minutes until softened.

3. Once the sweet potatoes is cooked, add it to the pan with the drained black beans and hot sauce.

4. Lightly stir together the ingredients, ensuring the vegetables and beans are evenly coated in the sauce.

5. Once the mixture is combined, and when the beans are heated through, remove from the heat.

6. Divide the bean mixture equally between the two tortilla wraps, top with the sliced avocado and fold up the wraps. Enjoy!

BBQ CHILLI BEANS ON TOAST

Serves 1

Beans on toast is definitely a staple in my diet! Spice this dish up by making beans with a BBQ kick.

Ingredients

2 slices bread, for toasting
1 tin chickpeas, drained and rinsed
1 x 400g tin chopped tomatoes
1 tin three-bean salad, drained and rinsed
1 pepper
1 onion
2 garlic cloves
1 tbsp BBQ sauce
1 tsp cumin
1 tsp coriander
1 tsp ginger
1 tsp chilli powder
1 tsp turmeric
1 tsp black pepper
1 tsp salt

1. Grease and preheat a non-stick frying pan over a medium heat.

2. Finely chop the garlic, onion and pepper and add to the pan.

3. Cook for 2 to 5 minutes before adding all the seasoning and spices, making sure the vegetables are evenly coated.

4. Add in the chickpeas, beans and chopped tomatoes to the vegetables.

5. Bring to the boil and add the BBQ sauce, then reduce the heat and leave to simmer for 10 minutes.

6. Toast your bread, then remove the beans from the heat and add to your toast.

RED LENTIL AND CARROT
BREAKFAST FRITTERS

Makes 6

This is a little bit like having a burger for breakfast – except perhaps a tad more acceptable and healthier!
I would serve around three hearty fritters per person, dipped into a spicy yogurt sauce.

Ingredients

6 tbsp red lentil flour
60g red lentils
2 sweet potatoes, grated
1 carrot, grated
1 bunch spring onions, chopped
½ white onion, finely chopped
2 garlic cloves, chopped
1 tsp paprika
1 tsp cumin
1 tsp black pepper
1 tsp salt
1 tbsp olive oil
large handful of coriander, chopped

For the dipping sauce

2 tbsp vegan soy plain yogurt
1 tbsp hot sauce
1 tsp chives, chopped

1. Preheat a non-stick frying pan over a medium heat and add the olive oil.

2. Add the sweet potato, chopped onion, grated garlic, spring onion and grated carrot to the pan and cook for 5 to 10 minutes until softened.

3. Meanwhile, in a separate pot, boil the red lentils until cooked through.

4. Add the cooked vegetable mix and cooked lentils to a food processor along with the flour, paprika, cumin, black pepper, coriander and salt then pulse together until combined. The mixture should stick together and have an easily mouldable consistency.

5. Using your hands, make six patties and place them back into the frying pan.

6. Cook each side evenly until each patty is golden brown.

7. While the patties are cooking, mix together the soy yogurt, hot sauce and chives.

8. Take the patties off the heat and serve with the dipping sauce.

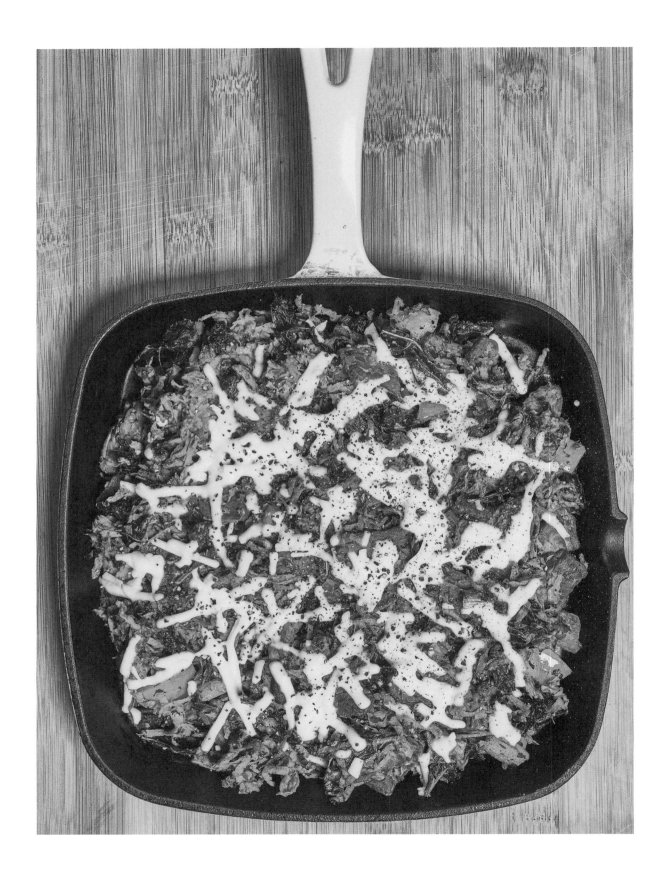

SWEET POTATO AND TEMPEH HASH

Serves 1–2

This is a delicious dish to serve up for breakfast: the combination of sweet potato and tempeh mixed with veggies is a great way to start the day.

Ingredients

2 sweet potatoes, grated with a cheese grater
200g tempeh, cut into 1-inch cubes
1 yellow pepper, cut into small chunks
½ white onion, diced
handful of kale, roughly chopped
2 tbsp olive oil
2 tbsp balsamic vinegar
1 tsp cumin
1 tsp paprika
1 tsp coriander
1 tsp black pepper
1 tsp salt
1 garlic clove, minced
sprinkle of vegan cheese, optional

1. Add the sweet potato, onion, garlic and pepper to a preheated frying pan and cook on a medium heat until soft.

2. Add the olive oil and the tempeh to the pan, stirring to combine all the ingredients.

3. Once the tempeh is cooked through, add the kale to the pan and sauté until it has wilted.

4. Add the spices, salt, pepper and the balsamic vinegar to the pan and cook for a further 2 minutes.

5. Serve with an optional sprinkling of vegan cheese.

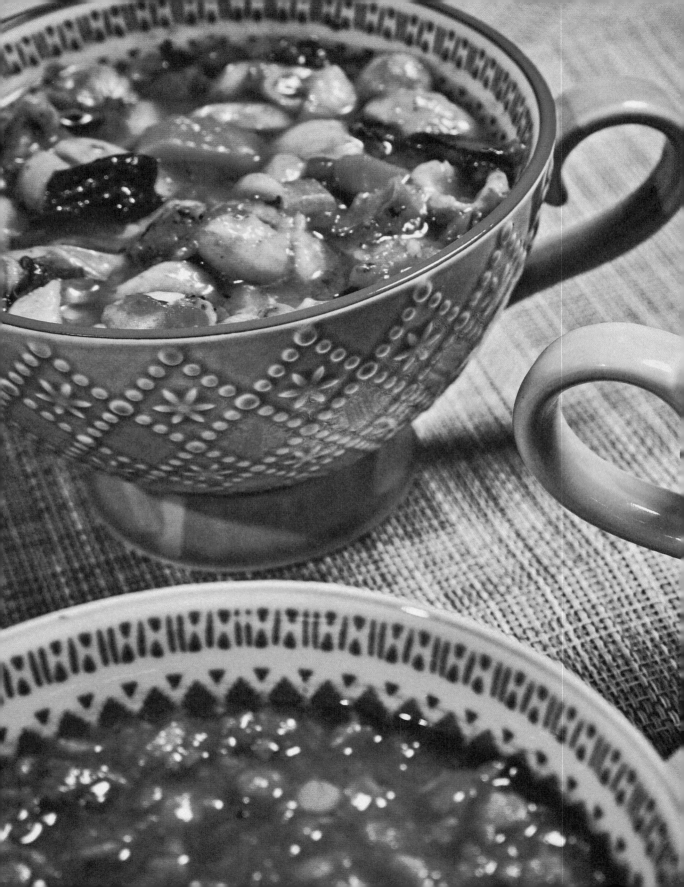

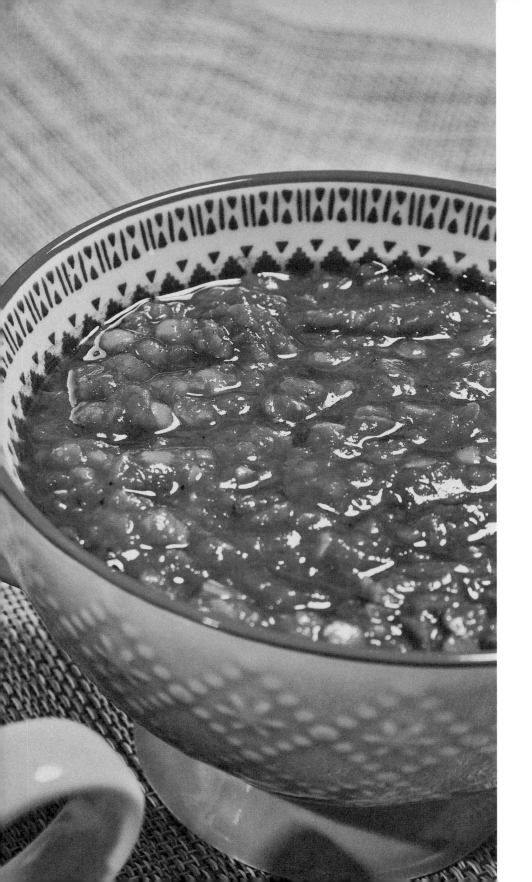

SOUPS

SOUPS

SPICED CARROT AND LENTIL SOUP

Serves 4

When winter hits Scotland, this is one of my go-to meals. I love hearty lentil dishes in the colder months and this soup is so quick and easy to make. It's also handy to make in large batches and keep in the fridge or freezer for your weekday lunches.

Ingredients

200g red split lentils
1 x 400g tin of chopped tomatoes
4 large carrots, chopped into small chunks
1 white onion, diced
3 garlic cloves, minced
1 litre of vegan stock
1 tbsp cumin
1 tbsp coriander
1 tsp turmeric
1 tbsp paprika
½ tbsp chilli powder
1 tbsp olive oil
salt and black pepper to taste

1. First add the olive oil to a large preheated saucepan or pot.

2. Add in the onion, garlic and carrot and cook over a medium heat until they begin to soften.

3. Stir in the cumin, coriander, turmeric, paprika and chilli powder.

4. Stir in the chopped tomatoes, lentils and stock, bring to the boil and then turn down the heat. Allow to simmer for 30 minutes or until the lentils have cooked through.

5. Add salt and pepper to taste.

6. Serve with warm bread.

MUM'S MINESTRONE

Serves 4

As shown in this recipe's name, my mum really does make a mean minestrone, so it was only fitting to add it to this book!

Ingredients

2 x 400g tins chopped tomatoes
1 x 400g tin of garden peas
50g pack of pasta
2 carrots, chopped
1 white onion, chopped
1 stalk celery, chopped
4 garlic cloves, minced
1 litre of vegan stock
1 tbsp dried parsley
1 tbsp dried basil
1 tbsp dried oregano
salt and black pepper to taste

1. In a preheated soup pot add the onion, celery, carrot and garlic and cook until softened.

2. Mix in the parsley, basil, oregano, salt and pepper and combine well.

3. Add the stock and bring to the boil for 10 minutes.

4. Add in the tomatoes, peas and pasta and simmer the soup for 10 to 15 minutes or until the pasta is cooked through.

5. Serve with warm bread.

DAD'S SCOTCH BROTH

Serves 4

This is the soup of my childhood. My dad used to make this potato and lentil-based soup every Christmas Eve and it was my favourite festive tradition. Serve alongside lots of warm bread and vegan butter!

Ingredients

4 large potatoes, cut into small chunks
3 carrots, cut into small chunks
1 bag of soup and broth mix containing
   barley, lentils and peas
1 celery stalk
1 white onion, diced
1 litre of vegan stock
1 tbsp olive oil
2 garlic cloves, minced
2 tbsp soy sauce
2 tbsp Dijon mustard
2 tbsp hot sauce
1 tbsp fresh rosemary, chopped
1 tbsp fresh thyme, chopped
1 lemon, juiced
salt and black pepper to taste

1. Preheat a soup pot over a medium heat and add the olive oil.

2. Add the carrot, celery, onion and garlic to the pot and sauté in the oil for a few minutes.

3. Stir in the potatoes then add the rosemary, thyme, salt and pepper, ensuring the vegetables are well mixed in with the herbs.

4. Add the soup and broth mix, stock, soy sauce, mustard, and hot sauce to the pan. Now bring to the boil.

5. Reduce to a simmer and leave to cook for 30 to 40 minutes until the lentils and potatoes are soft.

6. Top with lemon juice and extra black pepper then serve with warm bread.

TUSCAN KALE SOUP

Serves 4

This soup started out as one of those 'grab everything you have and throw it in a pot' type of meals. Thankfully it worked out and it's cheap and easy to make – perfect for a regular, weeknight meal.

Ingredients

200g brown lentils
3 tbsp tomato paste
2 x 400g tins of chopped tomatoes
2 carrots, diced
2 big handfuls kale, roughly chopped
1 celery stalk, diced
1 yellow onion, diced
4 cloves garlic, minced
1.3-1.5 litres of vegan stock
1 tsp dried thyme
1 tsp dried basil
1 tsp dried oregano
1 tsp salt
pinch of red pepper flakes

1. Add the onion, carrots, celery and garlic to a large preheated saucepan or soup pot and cook on a medium heat until the vegetables begin to soften. Add splashes of water if they start to stick to the pan.

2. Stir in the thyme, basil, oregano, tomato paste, salt and red pepper flakes.

3. Stir in the chopped tomatoes, stock and lentils, bring to the boil and simmer on low heat for 20 to 30 minutes until the lentils are cooked through.

4. Mix in the kale around 5 minutes before you're ready to serve. Allow it to wilt before taking the soup off the heat.

5. Serve by itself or with crusty bread.

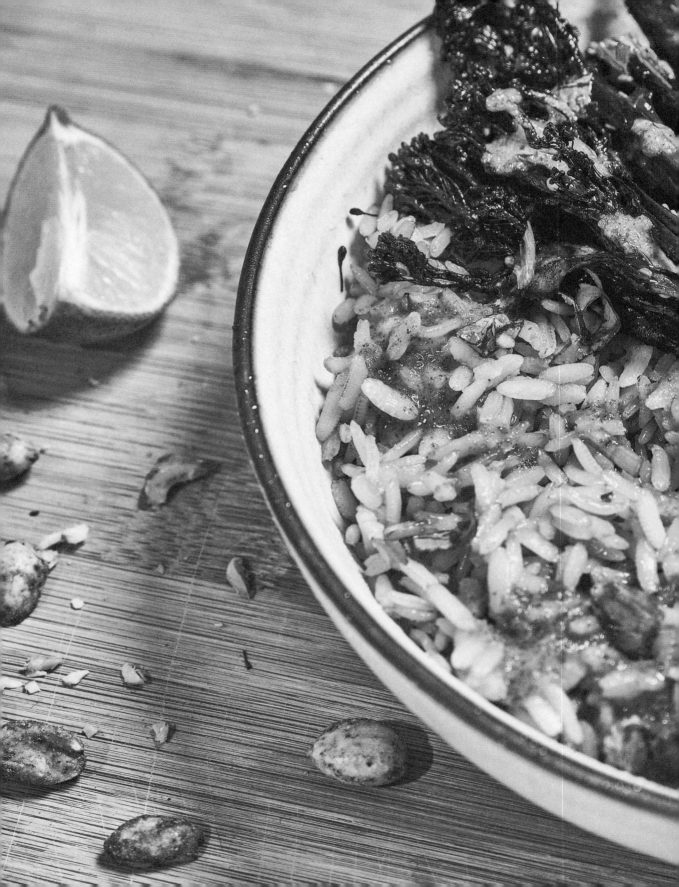

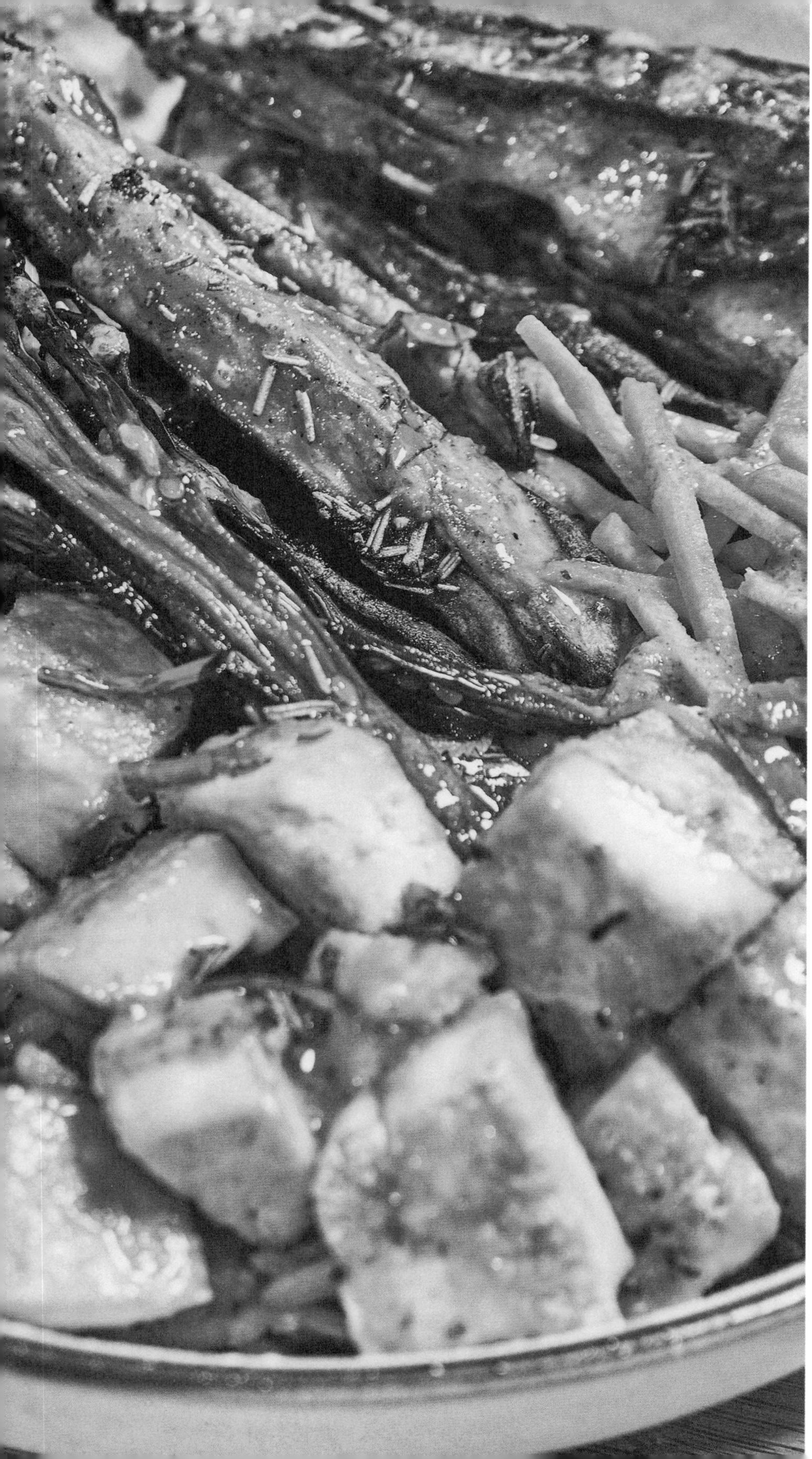

NOURISH BOWLS

NOURISH BOWLS

PEANUT BUTTER BUDDHA BOWL

Serves 1

*A mix of autumnal flavours brings this bowl together for a warming,
hearty meal that will leave you feeling full and satisfied.*

Ingredients

200g tofu
1 sweet potato
100g broccoli, cut into small florets
1 large carrot, peeled and chopped into
  cubes
1 pak choi, loosely chopped
1 tin chickpeas, drained and rinsed

For the dressing

2 tbsp powdered peanut butter or regular
  peanut butter
2 tbsp maple syrup
2 tbsp soy sauce
1 garlic clove, minced

1. First cut the sweet potato into 1-inch cubes,
    then either boil or steam until cooked
    through.

2. Drain and pat dry the tofu to remove excess
    moisture, then cut into cubes.

3. Add the tofu to a preheated frying pan and
    cook until golden.

4. Add the chickpeas to the tofu, warming
    them through before removing the tofu and
    the chickpeas from the pan and setting to
    one side.

5. Add the broccoli, carrot and pak choi to the
    pan and sauté until cooked through.

6. Add the vegetables, tofu and chickpea mix,
    and the sweet potato to your bowl.

7. For the dressing, mix together the peanut
    butter, maple syrup, garlic and soy sauce, or
    blend until smooth, and pour over the bowl.

KUNG PAO BUDDHA BOWL

Serves 1

Bursting with flavour, this quinoa-based bowl is quick and easy to throw together and will get you through that afternoon slump. This is a simple recipe to prepare and make in big batches, so you can double or triple the quantities and store it in tubs to eat throughout the week.

Ingredients

100g quinoa (dry weight)
1 can chickpeas, drained and rinsed
1 large carrot, cut into matchsticks
½ broccoli, cut into florets
½ green onion, chopped

For the dressing

2 cloves garlic, minced
2 tbsp tamari or soy sauce
1 tbsp sriracha
1 tbsp chilli paste
1 tbsp maple syrup

1. Cook your quinoa according to the package instructions and set to one side.

2. Add in the carrots, broccoli and onion to a preheated, non-stick frying pan and sauté on a medium heat for 3 to 5 minutes until the veggies are lightly cooked but still crunchy.

3. Mix the garlic, tamari, sriracha, chilli paste and maple syrup together to form a sauce then add it to the pan along with the chickpeas.

4. Ensure the vegetables and chickpeas are evenly coated in the sauce, and that the chickpeas are warmed through, before removing the pan from the heat.

5. Add the quinoa to your bowl and top with the veggies and chickpeas.

NOURISH BOWLS

SOFRITA BOWL

Serves 1

Get your Mexican fast food fix with this blend of spicy tofu crumbs, black beans and guacamole piled on to a bed of rice and veggies. This is another recipe that is great as leftovers for the rest of the week.

Ingredients

200g tofu
60-90g rice, cooked (per person)
½ tin black beans, drained and rinsed
2 cloves garlic, minced
1 jalapeño or chilli, finely chopped
½ red onion, finely chopped
1 tbsp guacamole (page 126)
1 tbsp mild salsa (page 127)
½ lime, juiced
handful of shredded lettuce

1. Drain and press out the excess water from your tofu then crumble it with a fork so it looks like large breadcrumbs.

2. In a preheated, non-stick pan, cook the tofu, garlic, onion and chilli until the tofu starts to turn a golden-brown colour.

3. Add the black beans and salsa to the pan and stir to combine.

4. Remove from the heat, add the tofu mixture and rice to your bowl.

5. Top with the guacamole, shredded lettuce and a squeeze of lime juice.

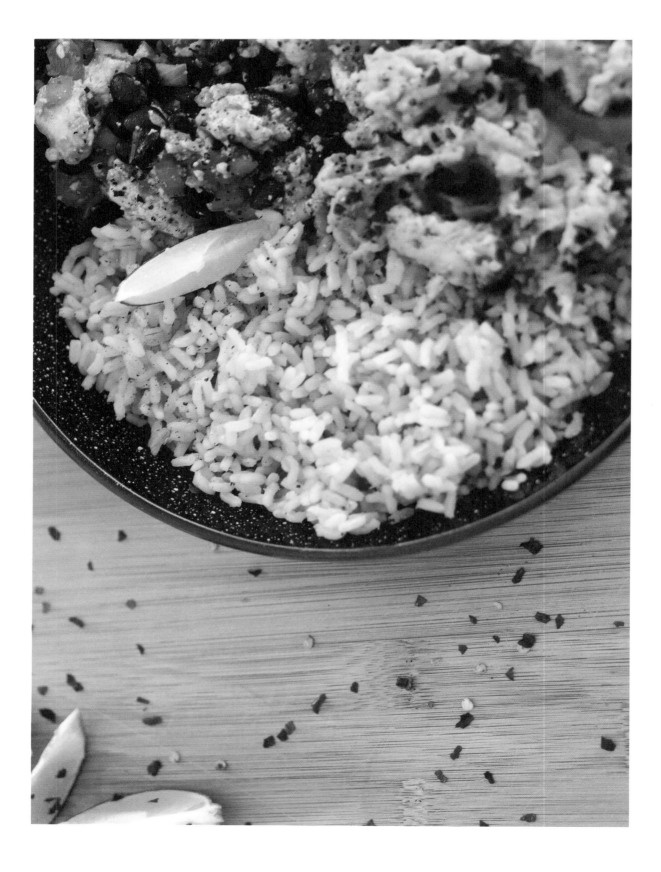

DECONSTRUCTED BURRITO BOWL

Serves 1

Grab a tortilla or two and wrap up the contents of this bowl for an on-the-go burrito or have it without bread for a lighter lunch option.

Ingredients

60-90g rice, cooked (per person)
½ tin black beans, drained and rinsed
½ tin kidney beans, drained and rinsed
½ yellow pepper, chopped into cubes
¼ red onion, diced
40g jalapeños
handful of fresh coriander
black pepper

Toppings

1 tbsp guacamole (page 126)
1 tbsp of salsa (page 127)
1 tbsp vegan mayo
1 lime, juiced

1. Add your pepper and onion to a preheated, non-stick pan and sauté until softened.

2. Add your beans and jalapeños to the pan along with the coriander and black pepper.

3. Layer your bowl with cooked rice, the vegetable mix, and the beans and jalapeños.

4. Top with salsa, guacamole and mayonnaise. Finish off with a squeeze of lime juice.

CLASSIC BODYBUILDERS' BOWL

Serves 1

Three main protein sources make up this protein-packed bowl, perfect as a post-workout meal to aid recovery and help you regain energy.

Ingredients

100g edamame beans
200g tempeh
100g tenderstem broccoli
1 serving cooked quinoa (approximately 90g)
2 handfuls of fresh spinach
tahini salad dressing (page 128)

1. Add the tempeh to a preheated, non-stick frying pan and cook either side until crispy.

2. Remove the tempeh from the pan and set to one side.

3. Add the broccoli to the same pan and cook for 2 to 3 minutes or until the desired texture is reached.

4. Add the spinach and cook with the broccoli until wilted.

5. Make up your bowl with the cooked quinoa, edamame beans, tempeh, and the spinach-broccoli. To serve liberally drizzle over some tahini salad dressing.

THAI PEANUT BOWL

Serves 1

This bowl is my personal favourite. Tangy Thai peanut sauce brings the tofu and vegetables to life and reminds me of my trip to Thailand – one of my all-time favourite holidays!

Ingredients

60-90g brown rice, cooked (per person)
100g tenderstem broccoli
200g tofu

For the sweet potato wedges

1 sweet potato
2 tsp rosemary
1 tsp garlic powder
1 tsp cinnamon

For the peanut sauce

½ tbsp soy sauce
½ tbsp maple syrup
1 tsp apple cider vinegar
1 tsp red Thai curry paste
30g peanut butter
60ml coconut milk

Toppings

1 carrot, shredded
handful of fresh coriander, roughly
    chopped
1 lime, juiced
salt and black pepper to taste

For the sweet potato wedges

1. Preheat your oven to 180°C and line a tray with non-stick baking paper.

2. Cut your sweet potato into long thin wedges and season with rosemary, garlic and cinnamon then add to the oven to cook for 20 to 30 minutes or until cooked through.

For the tofu

3. Drain and press the tofu to remove excess water and cut into cubes.

4. Add the tofu to a preheated, non-stick frying pan and cook until golden.

For the stir-fried broccoli

5. Add the tenderstem broccoli to a preheated, non-stick frying pan and fry until tender.

For the peanut sauce

6. Add the coconut milk, peanut butter, Thai curry paste, vinegar, soy sauce and maple syrup to a large bowl and mix well.

To combine

7. Add the cooked broccoli, tofu and sweet potato wedges to a bowl with the rice. Layer on the fresh carrot, coriander and a squeeze of lime juice.

8. Cover the bowl with drizzles of the peanut sauce and top with black pepper.

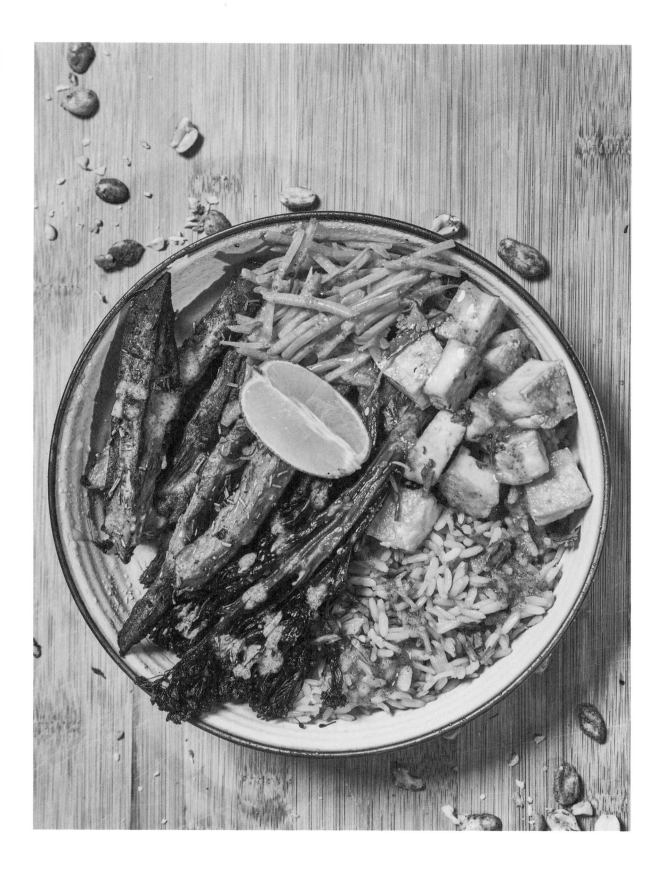

BAKED CHILLI TOFU NOODLE BOWL

Serves 1

*An easy weeknight meal that everyone can enjoy – just be sure to allow time
for your tofu to marinate in its lovely hot flavours.*

Ingredients

200g tofu
1 x 50g serving rice noodles
100g carrots, cut into matchsticks
100g tenderstem broccoli
100g sugar snap peas
1 spring onion, chopped

For the marinade sauce

4 tbsp soy sauce
1 tsp chilli flakes
½ tbsp maple syrup
½ tbsp sriracha hot sauce
½ tsp garlic powder

For the marinated tofu

1. Preheat the oven to 180°C and line a tray with baking paper.

2. Drain and remove the excess water from the tofu, then cut into thin slices.

3. Make the marinade sauce for the tofu by mixing together the soy sauce, maple syrup, hot sauce, chilli flakes and garlic powder in a large bowl.

4. Add the tofu slices to the sauce and marinate for at least 15 minutes.

5. Transfer the tofu to the baking tray and cook in the oven for 20 to 30 minutes or until golden brown, flipping the slices after 10 to 15 minutes to ensure the tofu is evenly baked.

For the stir fry

6. While the tofu is cooking, cook your rice noodles according to package instructions.

7. Stir fry the carrot, broccoli, sugar snap peas and spring onion in a wok, or large frying pan, for around 2 to 3 minutes until lightly cooked but still crunchy.

8. Add your cooked noodles to the wok, mix thoroughly, then add any leftover marinade sauce to the stir fry.

9. Remove from the work and top with the crispy tofu slices. Enjoy!

NOURISH BOWLS

SUMMER ROLLS SALAD BOWL

Serves 1

On my last visit to America, I stayed in a hotel that had a sushi counter right across the road. It was full of vegan options, and I spent ages in there every day picking out sushi to accompany my favourite rice paper rolls. The best part of the sushi, in my opinion, was the peanut sauce. As soon as I got back from America, I had to have a go at re-creating it. This dish is what I came up with.

Ingredients

200g tempeh
100g purple cabbage
5 sheets Vietnamese rice paper
2 small carrots
2 green onions
1 avocado
1 mango
½ cucumber
1 iceberg lettuce

For the peanut butter dipping sauce

60ml coconut milk
30g peanut butter
1 tsp red Thai curry paste
1 tsp apple cider vinegar
½ tbsp soy sauce
½ tbsp maple syrup
salt and black pepper to taste

For the peanut butter dipping sauce

1. Mix together the coconut milk, peanut butter, curry paste, vinegar, soy sauce, maple syrup, salt and black pepper.

2. Serve in a small, wide bowl to make the dipping process as easy as possible!

For the salad bowl

3. Cut the tempeh into strips and add it to a preheated, non-stick frying pan and cook for 2 to 3 minutes until golden.

4. Fill a large bowl with hot water and dip your rice paper in it for 15 seconds or less until it softens. Then remove from the water and set to one side. It will continue to soften while you add the filling.

5. Slice the cabbage, carrots, avocado, mango, cucumber and lettuce very finely into short strips.

6. Lay a piece of rice paper flat on your work surface.

7. Add small amounts of the vegetables, mango and tempeh to the edge of the roll closest to you, leaving a couple of centimetres free to wrap over the filling before starting to roll up the rice paper. Tuck in the edges of the roll as you go to ensure the filling doesn't fall out. Repeat with all five sheets of paper.

8. To serve, slice the rolls in half and dip in the peanut butter sauce.

BUILD YOUR OWN EPIC BOWL

Serves 1

Nourish bowls started with me initially just grabbing whatever I had in my cupboards and fridge and throwing it together to make a meal. Sometimes that's the best way and some of my favourite meals have been made by simply using what I had available. So, pick what you have at home from the list below and combine them to build your own epic bowl of goodness, perfect for your post-workout recovery lunch or dinner or just as a super quick option for your packed lunch tomorrow.

1. CARBOHYDRATE BASE: Choose one

- Brown rice
- White rice
- Quinoa
- Rice noodles
- Wholewheat noodles
- Soba noodles
- Pasta
- Lentil pasta
- Couscous

2. PROTEIN PUNCH: Choose one

- Tofu
- Tempeh
- Seitan
- Black beans
- White beans
- Mixed beans in water
- Kidney beans
- Lentils in water
- Red split lentils

3. VEGETABLES: Choose three

- Broccoli
- Carrot
- Green beans
- Courgettes
- Spinach
- Sweetcorn
- Pepper
- Onion
- Mushroom
- Potato
- Sweet potato
- Kale
- Lettuce

4. FATS: Choose one (a handful of nuts or a tbsp of seeds)

- Avocado
- Almonds
- Cashews
- Chia seeds
- Flax seeds
- Hemp seeds
- Peanuts
- Pecans
- Pine nuts
- Pumpkin seeds
- Sesame seeds

5. DRESSING: Choose one

- Guacamole (page 126)
- Hummus (page 126)
- Salsa (page 127)
- Tahini salad dressing (page 128)
- Avocado and herb salad dressing (page 128)
- Easy peasy pesto (page 128)
- Soy sauce
- Teriyaki sauce

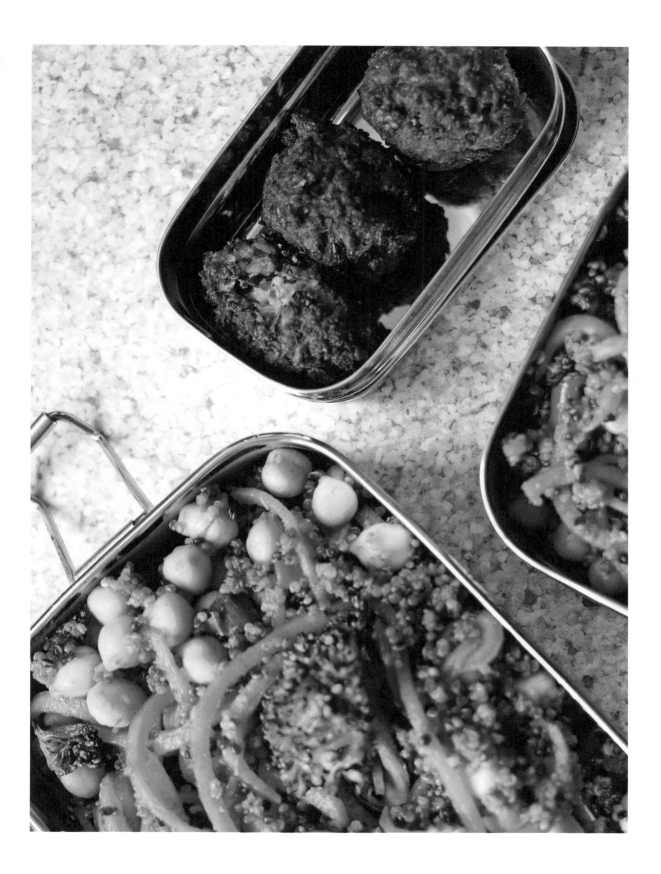

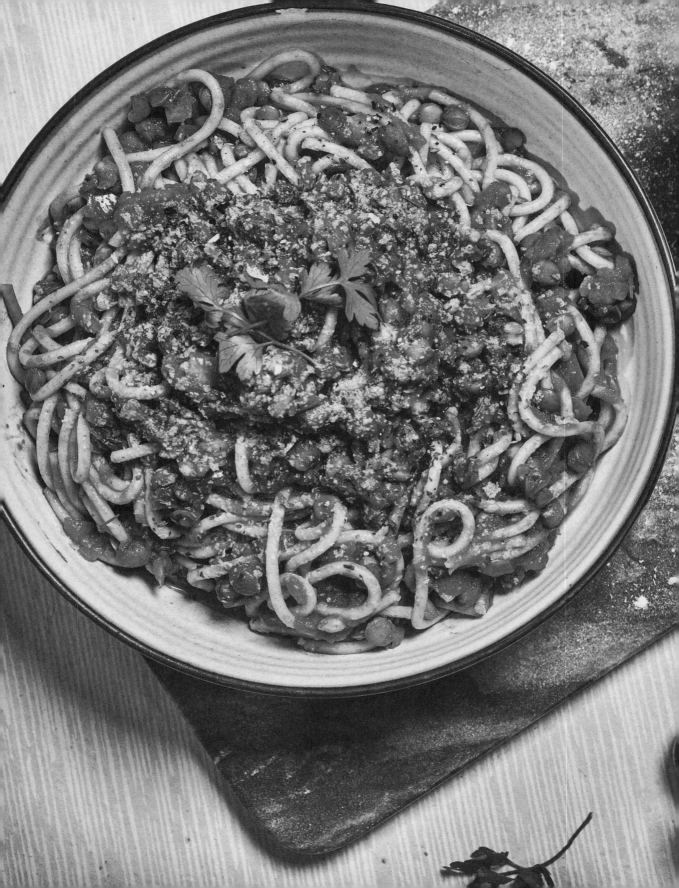

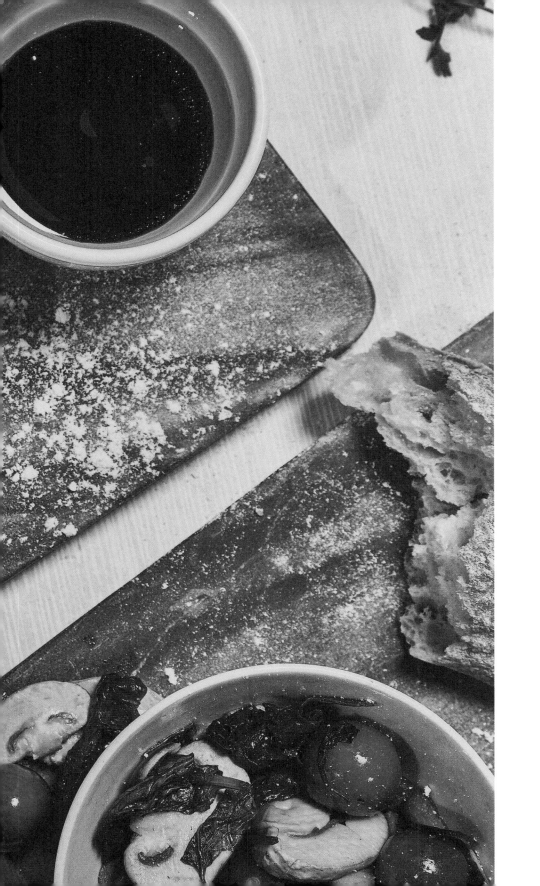

MAINS

FROM BOISTEROUS BURGERS TO CURRIES & BIG BOWLS

I can guarantee that every person has had at least one cooking fail in their life, but when I think back to the story I'm about to tell you, I'm amazed that I've come this far! As I've said, there is no need to overcomplicate healthy eating – my experience with cauliflower crust pizza is an example of this. Around six years ago, I wanted to make me and my now-husband, Marco, a super healthy pizza from cauliflower. I had just gone vegan and was eager to prove just how delicious the food could be.

What I didn't realise was you had to squeeze all the moisture out of the cauliflower before using it as a flour – that's where I went wrong and, unsurprisingly, it was an epic fail. The 'pizza' came out of the oven and instead of the beautiful, healthy pizza I'd had in mind, it was a sloppy plate of mushy wet cauliflower, decorated with tomato sauce and vegetables. Marco must have really liked me as he sat down and started eating it. Needless to say, I snatched it away and tossed it in the bin.

So, take it from me, you don't have to hunt the corners of the internet for an extravagant recipe just because you're vegan. Stick to the basics and you'll never have to face soggy cauliflower. The following main meals have got you covered.

MAINS

CHIPOTLE BLACK BEAN BURGERS

Serves 4

Have you ever been in a bit of a pickle where you can't decide between Mexican food or a juicy veggie burger? I can never choose between them, so I made a combination of the two! This burger is packed with Mexican-style black beans and rice and spiced up with jalapeños and chipotle sauce – making it a perfect Mexican-style veggie burger. This recipe makes four large burger patties so you can share with your family and friends or save them as leftovers for the rest of the week.

Ingredients

4 large sundried tomatoes, with the oil
1 tin black beans, drained and rinsed
200g brown rice, cooked
30g of oats or plain flour
40g of jalapeños (more or less depending on your preference)
¼ red onion
2 tbsp chipotle sauce
2 garlic cloves
1 tbsp paprika
1 lime, juiced

To serve

burger buns
lettuce leaves
vegan mayonnaise
extra jalapeños

1. Preheat your oven to 180°C and line a tray with baking paper.

2. In a food processor, combine the black beans, rice, oats or flour, sun dried tomatoes, jalapeños, lime juice, paprika, chipotle sauce, garlic and red onion and pulse until a loose, sticky mixture is formed.

3. Using your hands, make 4 patties. Don't worry if the mixture is still a little chunky, it'll just add to the overall texture.

4. Place the four patties onto the lined baking tray and bake in the oven for 30 minutes, turning the burgers over after 15 minutes to ensure they are evenly cooked.

5. Add the burgers to the buns, layering in the lettuce leaves, tomato, extra onion, jalapeños and topping with vegan mayonnaise.

PROTEIN-PACKED BURRITO

Serves 1–2

*In my humble opinion, few things in life beat wrapping up all your favourite foods in one giant tortilla –
comfort food at its best, great for lunch and dinner and perfect when you're out and about, too.*

Ingredients

2 tortillas
1 red bell pepper, sliced
100g brown rice, cooked
1 tin black beans in water, drained
    and rinsed
60g pickled red cabbage, chopped
    into long slices
½ red onion, diced
75g sweetcorn
½ tbsp paprika
½ tbsp cumin
½ tbsp chilli powder
40g jalapeños or chillies
guacamole (page 126)

1. Add the onion, pepper, black beans, sweetcorn and jalapeños to a preheated, non-stick pan and fry for 2 to 3 minutes until lightly cooked but still a little crunchy.

2. Add the paprika, cumin and chilli powder to the pan and mix well, ensuring the beans and vegetables are evenly coated in the spices.

3. Layer your tortilla with cooked rice, vegetable black bean mix, pickled red cabbage and a big dollop of guacamole.

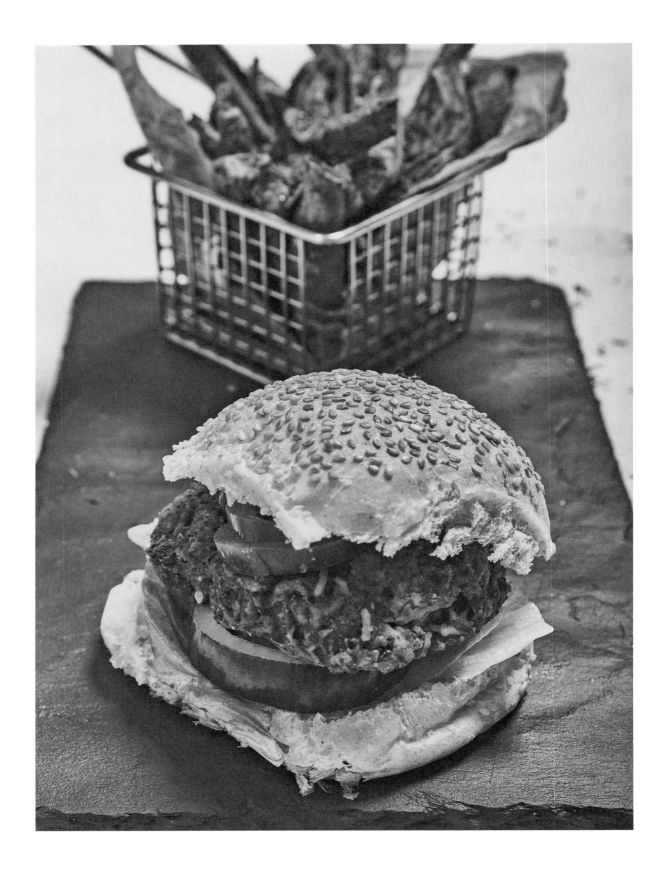

JALAPEÑO, LIME AND CHICKPEA BURGERS

Serves 4

I love this hearty burger patty with a salad or with some homemade fries. Like the black bean burgers, these last well in the fridge for up to three days and are also great in a nourish bowl or wrap.

Ingredients

1 x 240g tin of chickpeas, drained
  and rinsed
½ block tofu (approx. 150g)
½ red onion
60g jalapeños
30g oats or plain flour
1 tbsp paprika
1 tsp cumin
1 tsp coriander
½ lime, juiced

For the sriracha mayonnaise

1 tbsp vegan mayonnaise
1 tsp sriracha

To serve

burger buns
lettuce leaves
chopped tomatoes
extra jalapeños

1. Preheat your oven to 180°C and line a tray with baking paper.

2. Add the chickpeas, tofu, red onion, jalapeños, flour, paprika, cumin, coriander, lime to a food processor and pulse until the ingredients combine to form a loose 'dough'.

3. Using your hands, make four patties.

4. Place the 4 patties onto the tray and bake in the oven for 30 minutes, turning the burgers after 15 minutes to ensure they're cooked evenly.

5. Make the sriracha mayo by simply mixing together the sriracha hot sauce and mayonnaise.

6. Once the burgers are cooked, add the burgers to the buns, layering in the lettuce leaves, tomato, extra onion, jalapeños and topping with sriracha mayonnaise.

MAINS

AVOCADO PASTA WITH TEMPEH

Serves 1

The combination of avocado and hummus makes a creamy rich base for this pasta dish, while the basil and lemon fill it with flavour.

Ingredients

100g penne pasta
1 block tempeh
40g sundried tomatoes

For the sauce

100g hummus
1 ripe avocado
2 garlic cloves
1 lemon, juiced
1 tbsp olive oil
2 chillies (optional)
salt and black pepper to taste
handful of basil leaves

1. First cook the pasta and the tempeh following the pack instructions.

2. While the pasta and tempeh are cooking, use a blender or food processor to combine the avocado, hummus, garlic, lemon, basil leaves, oil, chilli, salt and pepper to create a thick, creamy sauce. Add a dash of water if it seems too thick.

3. Once the pasta and tempeh have cooked, add to a large serving bowl (depending on how many people you're serving), and stir in the avocado hummus sauce and the sundried tomatoes.

4. Serve topped with extra black pepper.

MAINS

TOFU CHICKPEA MASALA

Serves 2

*I love the tangy lemon flavour in this curry – it really brings it to life
and makes it both refreshing and delicious.*

Ingredients

60-90g rice (per person)
1 block tofu
1 can chickpeas, drained and rinsed
1 tin chopped tomatoes
1 white onion, diced
3 garlic cloves, minced
2-inch piece of ginger, finely chopped
2 chillies (optional), chopped
1 lemon
1 tbsp turmeric
1 tbsp garam masala
1 tbsp curry powder
1 tbsp cumin
1 tbsp coriander
1 tbsp black pepper
handful of spinach leaves

1. Cook your rice, following the pack instructions.

2. While the rice is cooking, drain and remove the excess water from the tofu and cut into cubes.

3. Add the tofu to a preheated, non-stick frying pan and cook for a few minutes on a medium heat until the tofu is a golden colour.

4. Blend the onion with the garlic, ginger and chillies and add to the pan. Cook for a further few minutes until the onions begin to soften.

5. Stir in the turmeric, garam masala, curry powder, cumin, coriander and pepper, adding splashes of water to ensure the spices don't stick to the pan.

6. Stir in the chopped tomatoes, chickpeas, a large squeeze of lemon juice and the spinach, bring to the boil and then turn down to heat. Allow to simmer for 15 to 20 minutes to infuse the flavours.

7. Remove from the heat and serve with the rice and top with an optional squeeze of lemon juice.

CHICKPEA FALAFELS

Makes 8–10

Falafel is like hummus, a vegan staple. If I think of vegan food, I think of falafel. Add these delicious falafels to pitta breads, wraps or salads or serve with dipping sauce as a starter or side.

Ingredients

1 tin chickpeas, drained and rinsed
40g plain flour
1 white onion, diced
4 garlic cloves
2 tbsp nutritional yeast
1 large handful fresh parsley
½ tbsp cumin
½ tbsp coriander
½ tbsp cayenne powder
½ lemon, juiced
salt and black pepper

1. Preheat the oven at 180°C and line a baking tray with baking paper.

2. Blend all of the ingredients in a food processor or blender to form a chunky dough.

3. Form 8 to 10 balls with the dough and place on the lined tray.

4. Drizzle the falafels with a little olive oil before cooking in the oven for 20 to 25 minutes until they turn a golden brown.

MAINS

78

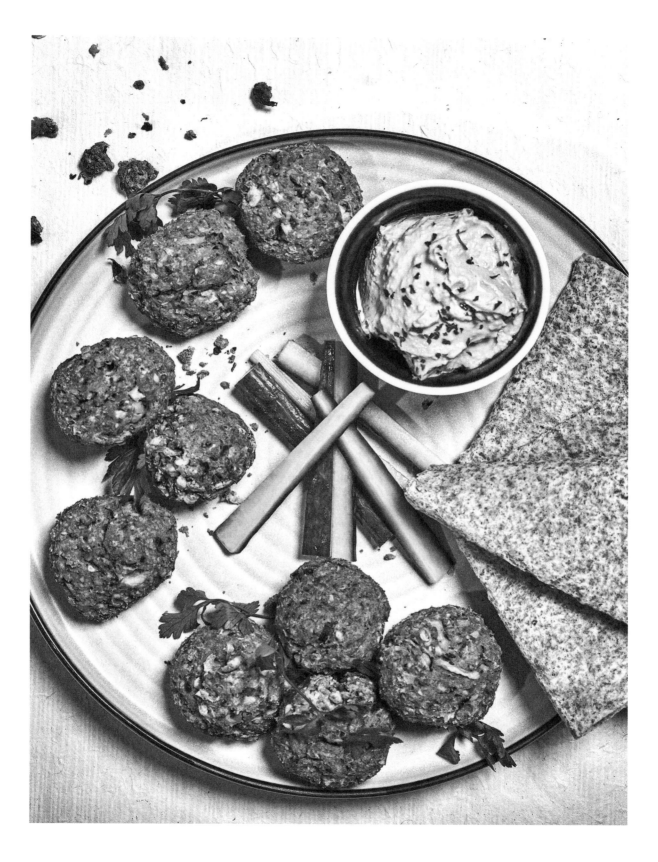

SESAME ORANGE SEITAN STIR FRY

Serves 1–2

A vegan twist on the popular Chinese Orange Chicken dish. Here, the chicken is replaced with seitan – I love using seitan in these types of dishes as it's healthy and easy to cook, while also soaking up loads of flavour and providing protein.

Ingredients

60-90g rice (per person)
200g green beans
200g of seitan
1 tbsp sesame seeds

For the sauce

2 cloves garlic, minced
2 tbsp soy sauce
1 tbsp white wine vinegar
1 tbsp maple syrup
1 tbsp tomato ketchup
1 tbsp sweet chilli sauce
1 orange, zested

1. Cook your rice according to package instructions.

2. While the rice is cooking, add the seitan to a preheated, non-stick pan and cook following the pack instructions.

3. Steam the green beans in a separate pan or in the microwave and add to the seitan.

4. Mix together the sauce ingredients then stir the sauce into the cooked seitan and green beans.

5. Serve with the rice and top with some extra sesame seeds.

MAINS

CURRIED TEMPEH WRAP

Serves 2

This wrap is great for on-the-go lunches. I always make a couple in advance and keep them in the fridge so I can easily grab one as I'm heading out the door.

Ingredients

2 wholemeal wraps
1 block tempeh
1 tin chickpeas
½ cauliflower, cut into bite-sized pieces
½ small white onion, chopped
2 cloves garlic, minced
2 tbsp fresh coriander, chopped
1 tbsp curry powder
½ tsp ground cumin
½ tsp mustard
1 tsp hot sauce
1 tsp lime juice
black pepper to taste

To serve

40g pickled cabbage
handful of lettuce leaves
2 tbsp plain vegan yogurt

1. Lightly steam the cauliflower for 5 minutes.

2. Preheat a non-stick frying pan over a medium/high heat, add the onion and cook until softened.

3. Add in the tempeh and cook for 2 to 3 minutes.

4. Stir in the garlic, curry powder, cumin and mustard.

5. Add the hot sauce, black pepper (optional), chickpeas and cauliflower to the pan and cook until the chickpeas are heated through.

6. Remove from the heat and stir in the lime juice and coriander.

7. To serve, lay the wraps out on your work surface or on a plate, divide the cauliflower tempeh mix between the two and top with the lettuce, pickled cabbage and yogurt before folding up the wraps.

MAINS

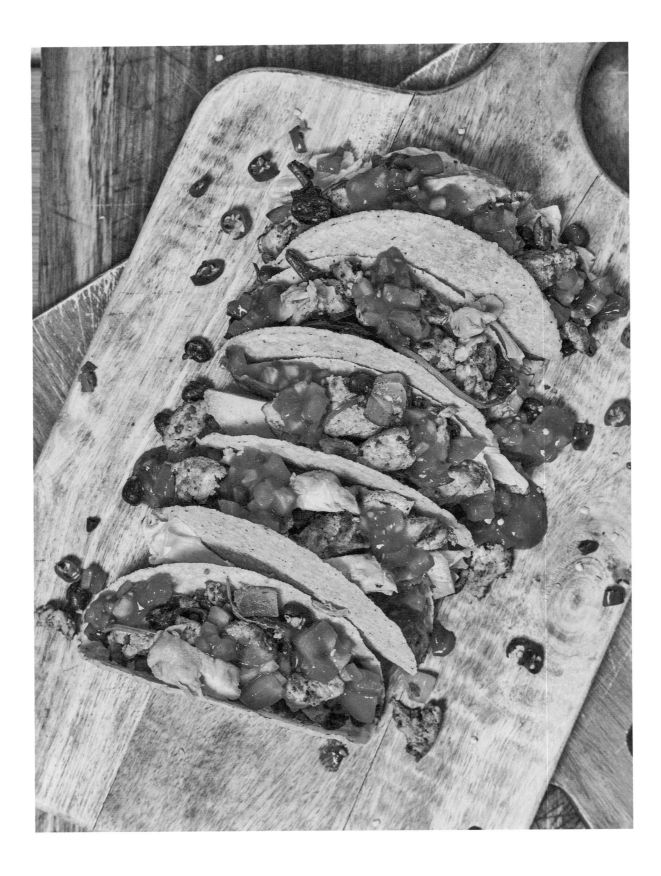

SCRAMBLED TOFU AND BLACK BEAN TACOS

Serves 2

This recipe is like having breakfast for dinner. I love this combination of two of my favourite meals.

Ingredients

200g tofu
5-6 taco shells
½ red onion, diced
2 cloves garlic, minced
2 tbsp nutritional yeast
1 tin black beans, drained and rinsed
handful of spinach, roughly chopped

For the spicy sauce

1 tbsp soy sauce
1 tsp turmeric
1 tsp paprika
1 tsp black pepper
1 tsp salt
1 tsp chipotle powder

To serve

1 avocado, sliced
2 tbsp salsa (page 127)

1. First drain and pat dry your tofu to remove excess moisture.

2. In a preheated, non-stick pan, crumble your tofu into small chunks and cook for around 5 to 7 minutes until it starts to turn golden brown.

3. Add in the onion, spinach and garlic to the tofu and cook for another 5 minutes until they have softened.

4. To make the sauce, mix together the soy sauce, chipotle powder and the spices, and add to the pan – making sure the tofu and vegetables are evenly coated.

5. Add the black beans and nutritional yeast and stir well.

6. Assemble your tacos by adding the tofu scramble to your taco shells, then topping with slices of avocado and a spoonful of salsa.

MAINS

SWEET POTATO AND JACKFRUIT QUESADILLAS

Serves 2

Crispy tortillas stuffed with juicy jackfruit, sweetcorn and crispy sweet potato
all melted together with cheese . . . irrestistible!

Ingredients

pulled jackfruit, store bought (can
    be substituted with black beans)
4 large tortillas
1 sweet potato, chopped finely or
    grated
handful of spinach
½ red onion chopped
1 tin sweetcorn, drained
1 tin kidney beans, drained and
    rinsed
1 pack vegan mozzarella cheese
2 tsp olive oil
1 tsp smoked paprika
1 tsp chilli
2 tbsp salsa (page 127)
1 lime, juiced

1. Add a teaspoon of olive oil to a preheated, non-stick frying pan and cook the sweet potato and red onion on a medium heat for a few minutes until they start to soften.

2. Add in the paprika and chilli to the pan and stir well.

3. Then add the sweetcorn, beans, jackfruit and spinach to the pan, combining all the ingredients.

4. Remove from the pan, transfer to a bowl and set to one side.

5. Add another tsp of oil to the pan and evenly coat the base of the pan – this is important to ensure the tortillas do not stick.

6. Add a tortilla to the pan and add half of your mix to the centre of the tortilla, leaving a 2-inch gap between it and the outer edge of the tortilla.

7. Sprinkle the filling with your vegan cheese.

8. As the cheese melts, add another tortilla over the top, pressing down the edges so the two tortillas stick together, sealing the filling in.

9. When the underside of the tortilla is brown, carefully flip, adding a little more oil if necessary, and cook on the other side.

10. Once the tortillas are evenly cooked, remove from the pan and slice into 4 to 6 equal pieces.

11. Serve your quesadillas with salsa and a squeeze of lime juice.

MAINS

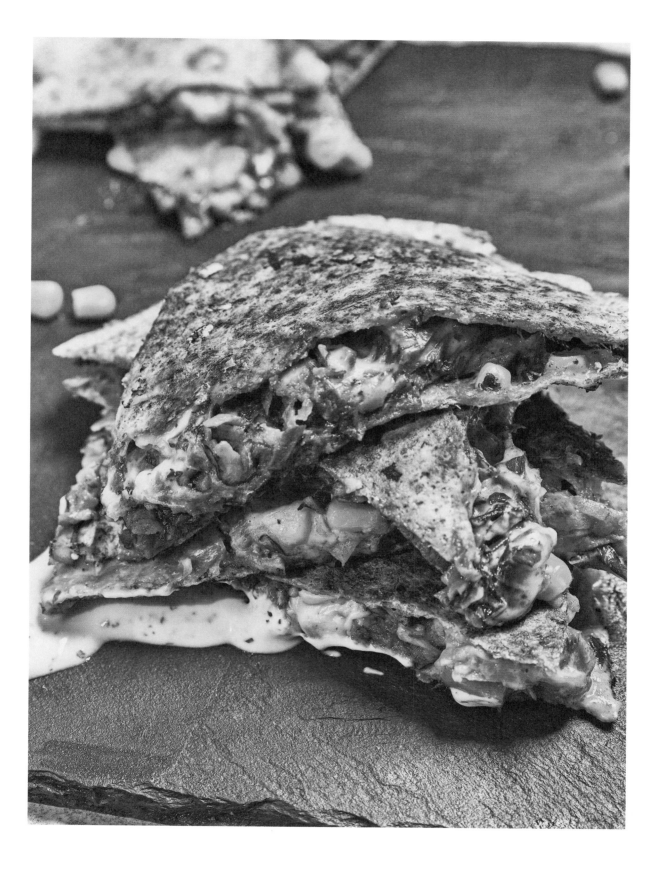

SCOTTISH COTTAGE PIE

Serves 4

Ah, cottage pie. A combination of my favourite foods: vegetables, lentils and chestnuts topped with creamy mashed potato then wrapped in puff pastry . . . so delicious! This recipe is a great replacement for a traditional Sunday roast; pair it with balsamic sprouts and sweet potato wedges and the meat-eaters will be envious.

Ingredients

150g chestnuts (store bought pre-cooked)
1 tin green lentils, drained and rinsed
1 celery stalk, chopped
1 carrot, finely chopped
1 onion, diced
230ml vegetable stock
2 garlic cloves, minced
1 tbsp cornstarch
1 tbsp vegetable oil
1 tsp thyme
1 tsp sage
salt and black pepper to taste
2 packets ready to use puff pastry sheets

For the mashed potato

3 large white potatoes, peeled
60ml almond milk
1 tbsp vegan butter
1 tsp cinnamon
1 tsp ginger
1 tsp salt
1 tsp black pepper

1. Preheat the oven at 180°C.

2. First cut the potatoes into chunks and steam them for 15 to 20 minutes until soft.

3. While the potatoes are cooking, add the vegetable oil to a preheated, non-stick pan.

4. Once the oil has warmed, add the onion, celery, carrot, chestnuts and garlic and cook for a few minutes until the vegetables start to soften.

5. Stir in the thyme, sage, salt and pepper, then add the green lentils and mix well.

6. Add the stock and cornstarch, bring to the boil before reducing to a simmer and cooking until most of the moisture has boiled off.

7. When the potatoes are cooked, drain them well then mash them, using a blender, potato-masher or fork, with the almond milk, butter and seasoning.

8. Roll out one sheet of the pastry and add to the base of a loaf tin lined with baking paper.

9. Add the lentil mix on to the pastry and flatten out evenly, top with the mashed potato and then close over the pie with another layer of pastry, sealing in the contents.

10. Cook for 30 to 40 minutes or until the pastry is golden.

11. To serve, lift the pie out of the tin using the baking paper lining.

THAI GREEN CURRY

Serves 1–2

This is my easy go-to dinner that takes less than 20 minutes to prep and throw together, perfect for any day of the week.

Ingredients

300ml carton coconut milk
200g tofu
120g chickpeas, drained and rinsed
100g broccoli
100g baby corn
100g red pepper, chopped
½ white onion, chopped
2 tbsp Thai green curry paste (fish free, vegan-friendly)
black pepper to taste

1. In a preheated pan add the vegetables and chickpeas and cook until softened.

2. Remove the vegetables and chickpeas from the pan and set aside.

3. Chop the tofu into chunks and cook either side until they start to turn brown.

4. Add the vegetables back in with the tofu and add the curry paste.

5. Add in the coconut milk and allow to simmer for 10 minutes.

6. Serve with rice.

MAINS

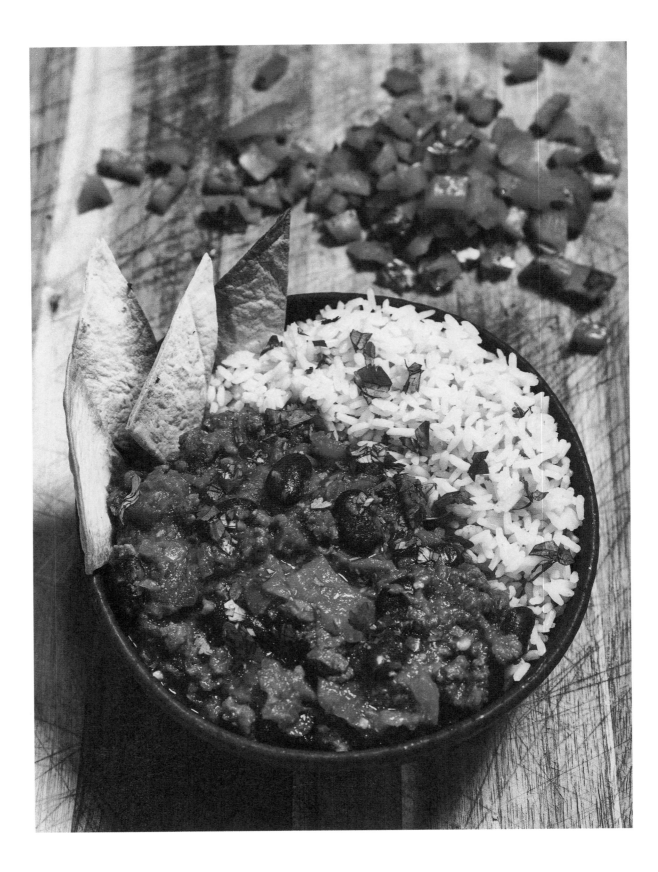

MEXICAN BEAN CHILLI

Serves 2–4

Everyone needs a basic chilli recipe. On top of baked potatoes or nachos, or served simply with a portion of rice, it's a go-to meal that can be enjoyed time and time again. Soya mince is a great meat alternative as it soaks up all the flavours of the chilli while also providing protein and texture to the meal.

Ingredients

1 x 400g tin of red kidney beans, drained and rinsed
200g frozen soya mince
2 tins chopped tomatoes
2 tbsp tomato paste
2 medium carrots, chopped into small cubes
2 red peppers, chopped into small cubes
2 celery stalks, chopped
3 cloves of garlic, minced
1 large onion, diced
1 tsp ground cumin
1 tsp chilli powder
1 tbsp smoked paprika
salt and pepper, to taste

1. Add the garlic, onion, celery, carrots and peppers to a preheated, non-stick pan and cook on a medium heat.

2. Once the vegetables have begun to soften, stir in the cumin, chilli powder, salt, pepper, smoked paprika, chopped tomatoes and tomato paste.

3. Separately cook the mince according to the package instructions and then add to the pan along with the kidney beans.

4. Allow to simmer for 10 to 15 minutes before serving.

SWEET POTATO MEXICAN-STYLE WRAPS

Serves 2

*These wraps are a total crowd pleaser! They're really quick and easy to make
and I love serving them to friends and family as they never disappoint.*

Ingredients

1 sweet potato, cut into 1-inch cubes
1 tin kidney beans, drained and rinsed
1 tin sweetcorn, drained
1 yellow pepper, finely sliced
1 red onion, diced
2 garlic cloves, minced
1 bunch fresh coriander, chopped
1 tsp cumin
1 tsp paprika
1 tsp coriander
1 tsp chilli powder
salt and pepper to taste

To serve

2 tbsp guacamole (page 126)
2 tbsp salsa (page 127)
2 limes, juiced
60-90g rice (per person)
4 tortillas, warmed

> If you're making these for a
> large group of people, why
> not do a 'make your own
> wrap' set-up and serve the
> potato mix, beans and rice
> and the variety of toppings
> in separate bowls so your
> guests can easily help
> themselves.

1. Cook your rice, following the pack instructions.

2. Assemble the rest of the wraps as the rice cooks. Create the spice mix by combining the salt, pepper, cumin, paprika, coriander and chilli powder.

3. Add the red onion, garlic, pepper and sweet potato to a preheated, non-stick frying pan and cook on a medium heat for a few minutes.

4. Stir the spice mix into the pan and continue cook until the potato has softened, adding splashes of water to prevent burning.

5. While the potato cooks, in a separate bowl, mix the kidney beans and sweetcorn together with the coriander and add to your cooked rice.

6. Pop the tortillas in the microwave or on a low heat in the oven to warm.

7. Once the potato mixture has cooked, remove your warm tortillas from the microwave/oven and lay them flat on your plate.

8. Layer your warm wraps with the potato mix, the bean and rice mix, salsa, guacamole and a squeeze of lime juice, then wrap up to serve.

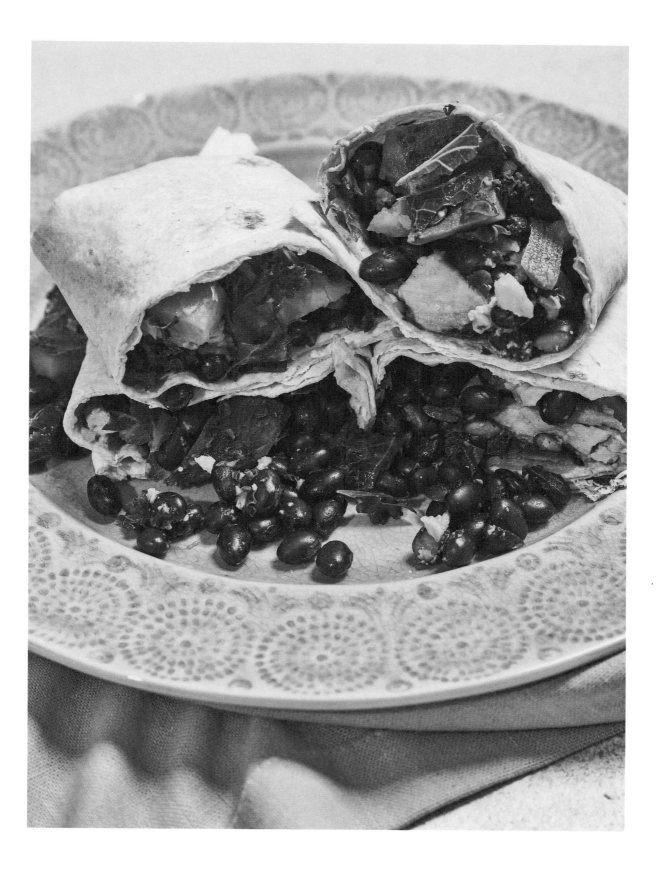

CREAMY GARLIC AND WHITE BEAN SPAGHETTI

Serves 1

This hearty and totally delicious dish is one of the meals I always choose,
especially when I need something really comforting.

Ingredients

250g silken tofu
100g spaghetti
100g broccoli, loosely chopped
100g frozen peas
½ tin butter beans, drained and rinsed
3 tbsp nutritional yeast
½ tbsp mustard
60ml almond milk
1 lemon, juiced

1. Add the tofu, lemon juice, almond milk, nutritional yeast and mustard to a blender or food processor and pulse to form a smooth mixture.

2. Cook your spaghetti, following the pack instructions.

3. While the spaghetti cooks, add the broccoli to a preheated, non-stick pan and sauté until cooked, add in the peas and beans until cooked through and then reduce the heat to keep warm.

4. Once the spaghetti is cooked, drain and then add to the broccoli, peas and beans.

5. Stir in the tofu sauce and remove from the heat.

6. Serve with lots of cracked black pepper

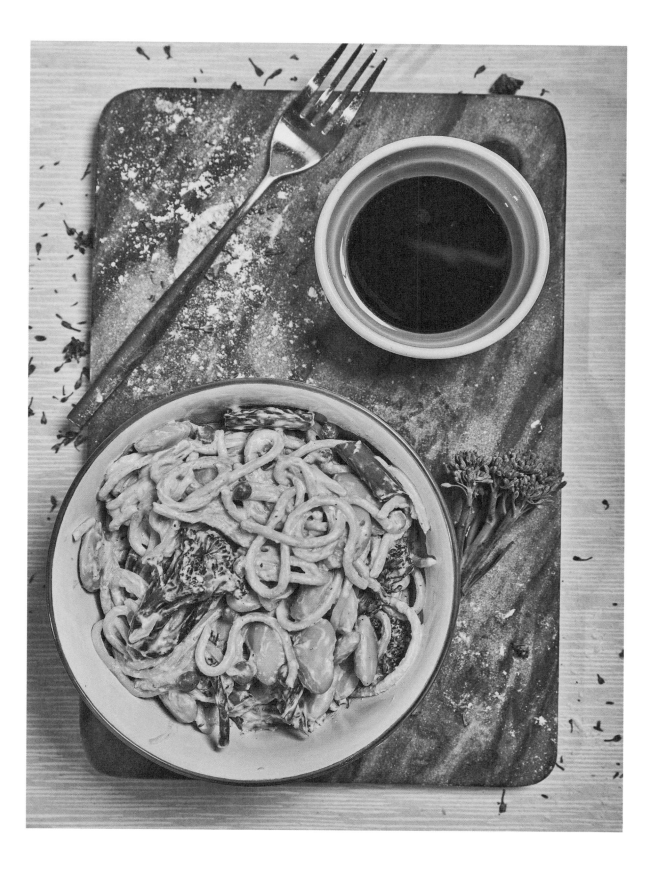

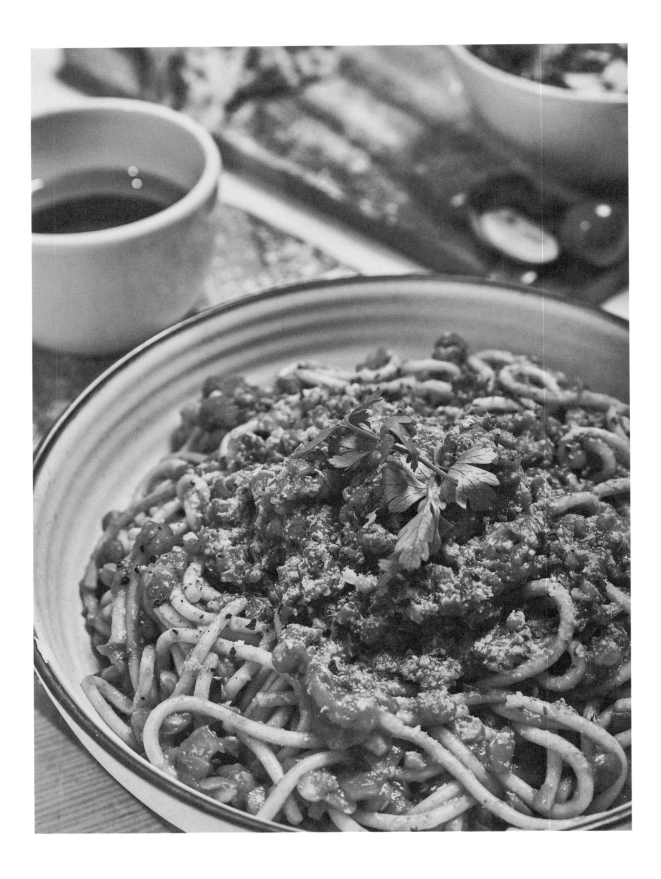

LENTIL BOLOGNESE

Serves 1

A vegan twist on the classic spaghetti Bolognese, using lentils for an additional protein punch. This is great recipe to serve to those who are sceptical about vegan food – it's a delicious vegan take on a classic, family meal and really highlights the fact that you can still eat your favourite foods on a plant-based diet.

Ingredients

100g spaghetti, dry weight
1 tin green lentils, drained and rinsed
1 yellow pepper, chopped
1 white onion, chopped
1 tin chopped tomatoes
2 garlic cloves, minced
2 red chillies, chopped
1 tbsp tomato paste
1 tbsp paprika
1 tbsp black pepper
½ tsp salt

1. Cook the spaghetti following the pack instructions.

2. Add the garlic, onion, chillies and yellow pepper to a preheated, non-stick saucepan and cook on a medium heat for 3 to 5 minutes.

3. Once these have cooked, stir in the chopped tomatoes, green lentils, tomato paste, paprika, black pepper and a sprinkle of salt, bring to the boil then turn down the heat and allow to simmer for 20 minutes.

4. Remove from the heat and serve with the cooked spaghetti.

LENTIL AND CHESTNUT LASAGNE

Serves 4

Before I switched to a plant-based diet, I was never very keen on lasagne – however, this lentil and chestnut variation really changed my mind. Heart-warming, full of delicious vegetables and with the meatiness of the lentils and chestnuts, it's the perfect dish for a cold night or a meal with family and friends.

Ingredients

15-20 vegan-friendly
    lasagne sheets
2 x 400g tin chopped
    tomatoes or passata
1 tin green lentils, drained
    and rinsed
150g mushrooms,
    chopped into small
    pieces
150g chestnuts
1 medium courgette,
    chopped into small
    pieces
1 large onion
2 tbsp tomato paste
3 garlic cloves, minced
1 litre vegan vegetable
    stock cube
1 tbsp olive oil
1 tbsp parsley
1 tbsp sage
1 tbsp thyme
1 bunch kale
salt and black pepper

For the 'cheese' sauce

800ml vegan milk (I use
    almond milk)
100g plain flour
3 tbsp olive oil
3 tbsp nutritional yeast
    flakes
salt and black pepper

1. Preheat the oven to 180°C.

2. In a food processor, pulse the onion, courgette, mushrooms, garlic, and chestnuts to form a chunky mixture.

3. Add this to a preheated, non-stick saucepan with the olive oil. Cook until the mixture begins to soften.

4. Stir in the lentils, herbs and the tomato paste, evenly coating the mixture in the herbs.

5. Add the chopped tomatoes, kale and stock, bring to boil and allow to simmer for 15 to 20 minutes. If the mixture looks too watery, stir in cornstarch to thicken.

6. In a separate pan, make the 'cheese' sauce. Warm the olive oil and then stir in the flour to form a crumbly mixture. Then stir in the almond milk, nutritional yeast, salt and pepper.

7. Whisk the sauce over a medium heat for around 5 to 10 minutes until it has thickened.

8. Once the vegetables and 'cheese' sauce are cooked, assemble the lasagne.

9. Add a layer of the lentil and chestnut mix to the base of a baking dish, then top it with a layer of lasagne sheets. Repeat this process once more.

10. Add another layer of the lentil and chestnut mix and this time top it with half the 'cheese' sauce. Top this sauce with a layer of lasagne sheets and then complete the dish with the rest of the 'cheese' sauce.

11. Bake the lasagne in the oven for 40 minutes until the lasagne sheets have cooked through.

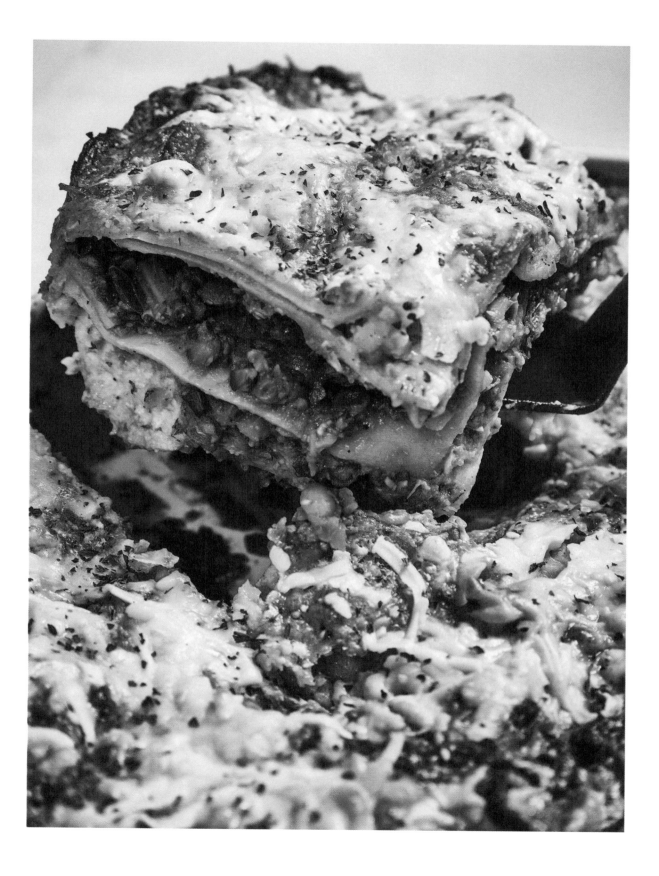

SPICY TOFU NOODLES

Serves 1–2

*Tofu is high in protein and low in saturated fat while also absorbing delicious flavours –
combined with the crunchy veggies, soft noodles and a sprinkle of chilli flakes, it's a great addition
to this dish. I love this meal as it's so tasty and super quick to make; it's also super easy to take
with you on the go, so I often double the recipe and have the leftovers for lunch the next day.*

Ingredients

100g or two nests of wholewheat noodles
300g tofu
100g mushrooms, chopped
100g broccoli
¼ medium cabbage, green or purple
2 carrots, cut into 'matchsticks'
4 scallions / spring onions
2 garlic cloves, minced
60ml soy sauce
1 tsp dark soy sauce
1 tbsp sriracha
2 tsp brown sugar
1 tsp rice vinegar
115ml water
chilli flakes to taste

1. Mix together the soy sauces, sriracha, brown sugar, vinegar and water.

2. Drain and remove the excess water from the tofu and cut into cubes.

3. Add the tofu and mushrooms to a preheated, non-stick pan and cook for a few minutes until the tofu is golden and mushrooms are juicy.

4. Sprinkle the tofu and mushrooms with chilli flakes, then remove from the pan and set to one side.

5. Add the broccoli, cabbage, carrots, scallions or spring onions and garlic to the pan and cook until softened.

6. Cook the noodles, following the pack instructions.

7. Stir the noodles and tofu into the pan with the vegetables before adding the sauce.

8. Ensure the sauce is evenly mixed before serving with an added sprinkle of chilli flakes.

TERIYAKI SOBA NOODLES

Serves 2

I have a love-hate relationship with mushrooms, but I encourage you, if you are the same, to give this dish a try. The roasted mushrooms are meaty and hearty and provide substance to this noodle dish.

Ingredients

1 serving of soba noodles
200g tenderstem broccoli, chopped
200g mushrooms, sliced
2 handfuls of kale, chopped
2 garlic cloves
2-inch piece of ginger, chopped
2 tbsp teriyaki sauce
1 tbsp maple syrup
1 tsp chilli flakes

Toppings

1 red chilli, sliced (optional)

1. Preheat your oven to 180ºC and line a baking tray with greaseproof paper.

2. Grate or mince the ginger and garlic together then add to a bowl with the teriyaki, chilli flakes and maple syrup. Mix well to create the teriyaki sauce.

3. Spread the sliced mushrooms out on the lined baking tray before coating in the sauce. Make sure the mushrooms are evenly covered for maximum flavour.

4. Roast the mushrooms in the oven for approximately 30 minutes, turning them after 15 minutes.

5. While the mushrooms are roasting, add the broccoli and kale to a preheated, non-stick frying pan and cook until softened.

6. Cook the soba noodles, following the pack instructions, and add to the pan.

7. After 30 minutes, remove the mushrooms from the oven and stir into the noodles, broccoli and kale.

8. Add any remaining teriyaki sauce to the dish before serving and topping with an optional sliced chilli.

MAINS

SPECIAL SUNDAY SAUSAGE CASSEROLE

Serves 3–4

There is something special about Sunday dinner. It's always been one of my favourite meals of the week and this hearty vegan sausage and bean casserole is one of best dishes to serve to end your weekend – and start your week – well. I love serving this with some warm bread as the ultimate comfort food.

Ingredients

6 vegan-friendly sausages
200ml vegan stock
150g mushrooms
2 carrots
2 garlic cloves, minced
1 white onion
1 tin butter beans, drained and rinsed
1 tin chopped tomatoes
1 tbsp tomato paste
1 tbsp paprika
1 tbsp dried mixed herbs
1 tbsp olive oil

1. Cook your sausages according to package instructions.

2. Add the oil to a preheated pan and cook the onion, garlic, mushrooms and carrots until softened.

3. Add in the tomato paste, herbs and spices and mix well.

4. Add in the sausages, butter beans, stock and chopped tomatoes and allow to simmer for 15 to 20 minutes.

5. Serve and enjoy with warm bread.

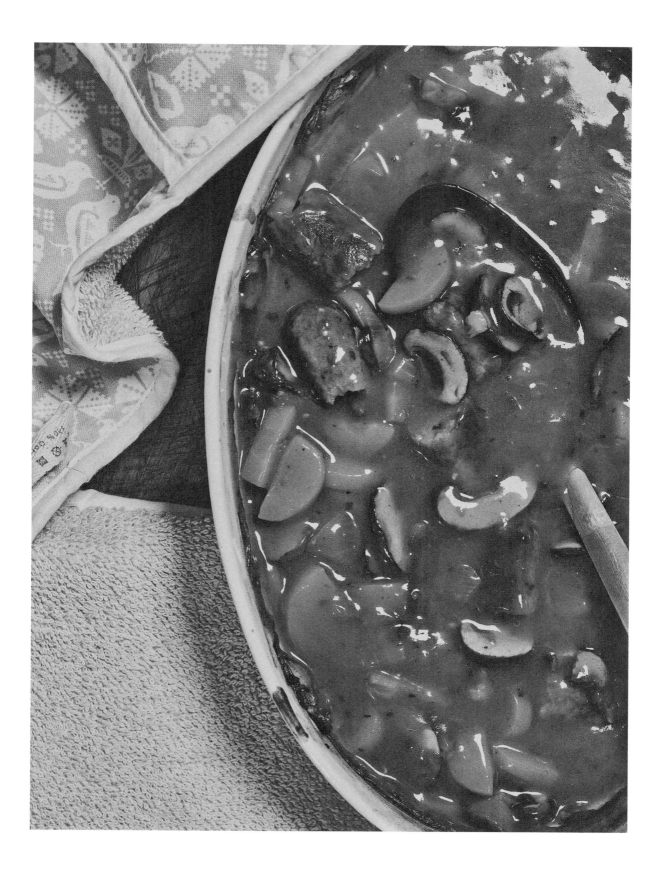

CHICKPEA, LENTIL AND SQUASH CURRY

Serves 2

A fragrant, autumnal curry that makes for a hearty meal – I love making this dish in the colder months as it's really warming and perfect for a cosy evening in.

Ingredients

100g brown rice (dry weight)
1 tin chickpeas, drained and rinsed
2 tins chopped tomatoes
250ml carton of coconut milk
100g red split lentils
1 white onion
2 tbsp tomato paste
2 handfuls of spinach
½ of a medium butternut squash or
   pumpkin
2 garlic cloves, minced
1 litre vegan stock
1 tsp turmeric
1 tsp black pepper
1 tsp paprika
1 tsp chilli powder

1. Start by setting the rice to cook, following the pack instructions.

2. Add the garlic and onion to a preheated, non-stick saucepan and cook over a medium heat.

3. Once the onion and garlic have begun to soften, stir in the tomato paste, chickpeas, turmeric, pepper, paprika and chilli powder.

4. Then add the lentils, coconut milk and stock to the pan, then leave to simmer for 20 to 30 minutes until the lentils have cooked through.

5. Add the spinach to the pan about 5 minutes before removing from the heat, letting it wilt.

6. Serve with the rice.

LENTIL AND SPLIT PEA CURRY

Serves 2

An easy go-to curry where you pretty much throw everything in a pan and leave it to cook itself for 30 minutes.
All you have to worry about is how many poppadoms you are going to eat while you wait . . .

Ingredients

300ml vegan stock
300ml carton of coconut milk
120g red lentils
120g yellow split peas
1 tin chopped tomatoes
2 tbsp tomato paste
1 yellow pepper, chopped
1 white onion, chopped
4 garlic cloves, minced
1 tbsp paprika
1 tbsp turmeric
1 tbsp cumin
1 tbsp coriander
1 tbsp hot curry powder
1 tbsp olive oil
salt and black pepper to taste

1. Add the oil to a preheated pan, then add the garlic, onion and yellow pepper and cook for few minutes until they start to soften.

2. Stir in the spices and tomato paste, with a few splashes of water to stop the spices from burning.

3. Next add in the lentils and split peas and mix well.

4. Add the coconut milk, stock and chopped tomatoes, bring to the boil and then reduce the heat and allow to simmer for 30 minutes until the lentils are cooked.

5. Serve with your choice of rice, naan bread or poppadoms.

MAINS

SRI LANKAN CASHEW AND POTATO CURRY

Serves 2

Cashew nuts in curries are my new addiction! They add texture and bite and are packed with iron, magnesium, zinc and copper. Curries are so simple to throw together, easy to make in large batches and are perfect as leftovers, too. If you are unable to eat cashew nuts, you can substitute them with sunflower seeds or leave them out altogether – the curry will still be delicious.

Ingredients

300ml carton coconut milk
300ml vegan stock
250g white potatoes, cut into cubes
200g green beans
1 tin green lentils, drained and rinsed
1 yellow pepper, sliced
1 white onion, diced
4 garlic cloves, minced
2 tbsp ginger puree
2 tbsp tikka powder
2 handfuls cashews
1 lemon, juiced
handful of spinach
handful of fresh coriander
salt and pepper to taste

1. Drain, pat dry and cut your tofu into cubes. Add to a preheated saucepan and cook either side until golden.

2. Remove the tofu from the pan and set to one side. To the same pan, add the onion, garlic, cashews, green beans and pepper and cook for a few minutes until the vegetables being to soften.

3. Add the tofu back into the pan with the vegetables. Stir in the tikka powder, ginger puree, salt and black pepper.

4. Add the coconut milk, stock, green lentils and lemon juice, bring to the boil then reduce the heat and allow to simmer for 15 to 20 minutes.

5. While the curry cooks, boil the potatoes in a separate pan for 15 to 20 minutes and add to the curry when cooked.

6. Stir in the spinach and allow it to wilt before serving with the fresh coriander.

MAINS

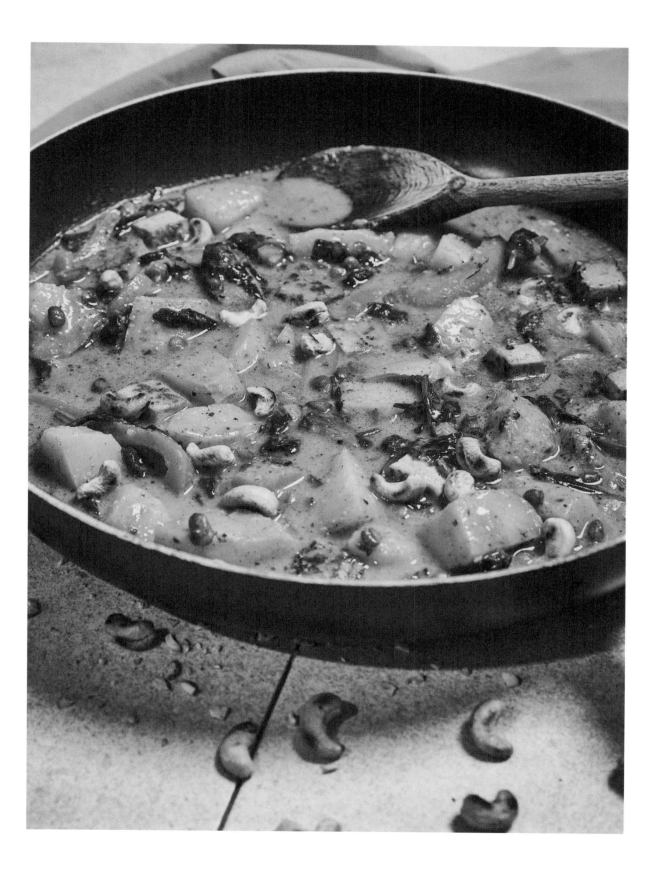

SEITAN AND CHICKPEA TAGINE

Serves 2

Seitan is a great meat replacement in dishes that need the texture and taste of a meaty component. This tagine combines chickpeas and seitan to make a hearty meal that will leave you feeling full and satisfied. This is fabulous served with fresh herbs, or with a warm flatbread or couscous.

Ingredients

500ml vegetable stock
100g seitan
1 tin chickpeas, drained and rinsed
1 tin chopped tomatoes
1 sweet potato, chopped into cubes
1 white onion, diced
2 garlic cloves, minced
1 tbsp olive oil
2-inch piece of fresh ginger, grated
1 tsp cumin seeds
1 tsp coriander seeds
1 tsp saffron
1 tsp ground ginger
1 tsp chilli flakes
1 tbsp maple syrup
½ tbsp cinnamon
handful of fresh coriander
handful of fresh parsley

1. Add the oil followed by the onion, garlic and fresh ginger to a preheated, non-stick pan and cook over a medium heat for a few minutes.

2. Stir in the cumin, coriander, cinnamon, saffron, ground ginger and chilli flakes.

3. Stir in the chopped tomatoes, maple syrup, seitan, sweet potato and vegetable stock, bring to the boil then reduce to a simmer until the potato has cooked through.

4. Once the potato has cooked, add the chickpeas and cook for a further 20 to 25 minutes, until the mixture is thick, and the sauce has turned a dark shade of red.

5. Stir in the fresh parsley and coriander and serve.

COCONUT TAHINI NOODLES

Serves 2

This rich and creamy dish is delicious, with the wholewheat noodles combining so well with crispy tofu and chunky veggies.

Ingredients

2 wholewheat noodle nests
300g tofu
100g broccoli, chopped
1 red pepper, chopped
1 onion, diced
100g sugar snap peas
2 cans of coconut milk
2 tbsp tahini (can also be substituted
   with a nut butter)
2 tsp sriracha
2 tbsp maple syrup
2 tbsp soy sauce
1 lime, juiced (to taste)

1. First juice the lime and mix together with the tahini, coconut milk, sriracha, sugar and soy sauce.

2. Drain and remove the excess water from the tofu and cut into cubes.

3. Cook the tofu in a preheated, non-stick frying pan or wok until it turns golden.

4. Add the broccoli, pepper, onion and peas to the pan and cook alongside the tofu until softened.

5. Cook the noodles, following the pack instructions, and then add to the pan.

6. Stir in the sauce and let it simmer for 10 minutes before serving.

MAINS

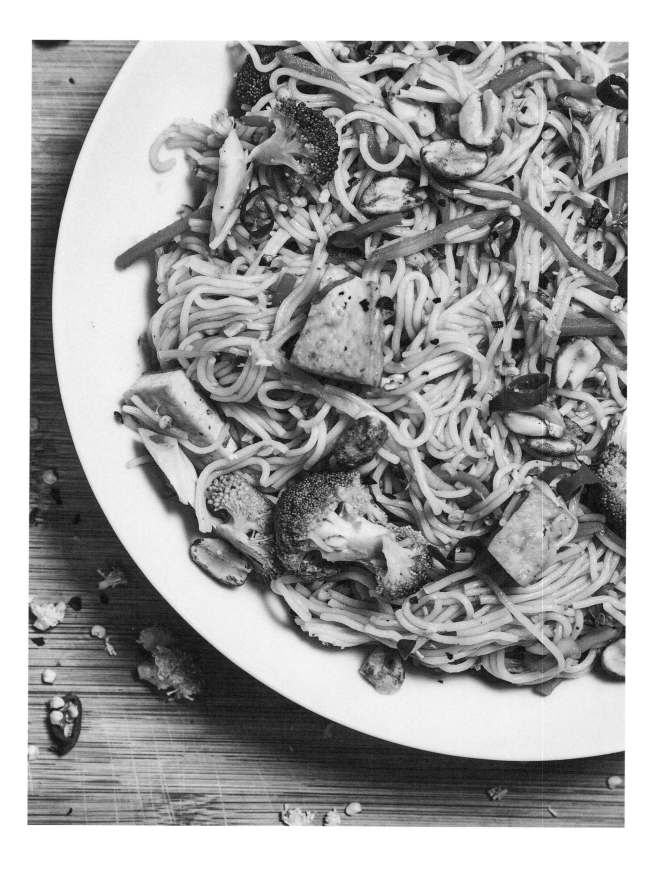

TOFU PAD THAI

Serves 1–2

I ordered this classic Thai dish nearly every day when I was in Thailand. The crunchy vegetables combined with soft noodles topped with crushed peanuts is a winning combination, and I had to recreate the experience once I'd arrived home.

Ingredients

200g tofu
100g rice noodles (dry weight)
120g bean sprouts
½ broccoli, chopped
2 carrots, chopped into matchsticks
2 spring onions , finely chopped
4 tbsp soy sauce
2 tbsp rice vinegar
2 tbsp pure maple syrup
2 tbsp fresh lime juice
1 tsp sriracha hot sauce
1 lime, juiced
1 lime, sliced to serve
1 tbsp crushed peanuts

1. Start by draining and removing the excess water from the tofu before cutting it into cubes.

2. Cook the tofu in a preheated, non-stick frying pan until golden.

3. Move the tofu to one side of the pan, then add and sauté the vegetables for a few minutes.

4. Cook the rice noodles following the pack instructions, then add them to the pan. Stir to combine.

5. Juice the lime and mix with the soy sauce, vinegar, maple syrup and sriracha, then add to the pan.

6. Ensure the Pad Thai is evenly covered in the sauce before removing from the pan and serving with the crushed peanuts and a slice of lime.

MAINS

LEMON TOFU FLATBREAD
WITH HERB YOGURT

Serves 1–2

When my favourite vegan restaurant in Glasgow discontinued my all-time favourite dish –
my beloved Bah Mi sandwich with a tofu flatbread – I was utterly heartbroken. However, it inspired
me to go away and make my own version, which I now think I prefer . . .

Ingredients

2 small wholewheat flatbreads of your
  choice
300g tofu
1 head cauliflower, cut into small florets
1 can chickpeas, drained and rinsed
plain soy yogurt or vegan crème fraîche if
  your supermarket sells it
1 lime, juiced
1 lemon, juiced
2 tbsp chives, chopped
1-2 tsp chilli powder
1 tsp garam masala
1 tsp cayenne pepper
salt and pepper to taste

1. Preheat the oven to 180°C and line two baking trays with baking paper.

2. Place the chickpeas and cauliflower florets in a bowl and stir in the chilli powder, garam masala, cayenne pepper, salt and black pepper. Make sure they are completely coated in the spices for maximum flavour.

3. Drain and remove excess water from the tofu and cut into thick, even slices.

4. Pour the lemon juice over the tofu then spread the lemon juice-infused slices onto one of the baking trays. Place the tray on the top shelf of the oven to cook.

5. Spread the chickpea and cauliflower mix over the second lined baking tray and place in the oven.

6. Cook both the tofu and the chickpea mix for 25 to 30 minutes until the tofu turns golden and the chickpeas crispy.

7. Meanwhile, in a separate bowl, mix the soy yogurt with the chives. Toast the pitta bread.

8. Once the tofu and chickpea and cauliflower mix have cooked, slice the pitta bread open to form 'pockets' and fill with sliced tofu and chickpea mix.

9. Serve with a dollop of yogurt and a squeeze of lime juice.

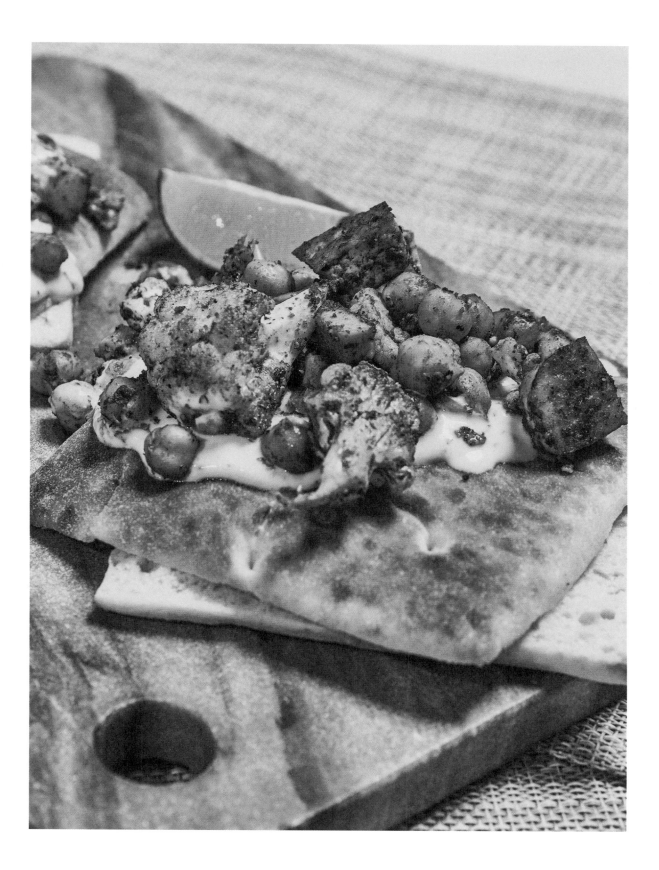

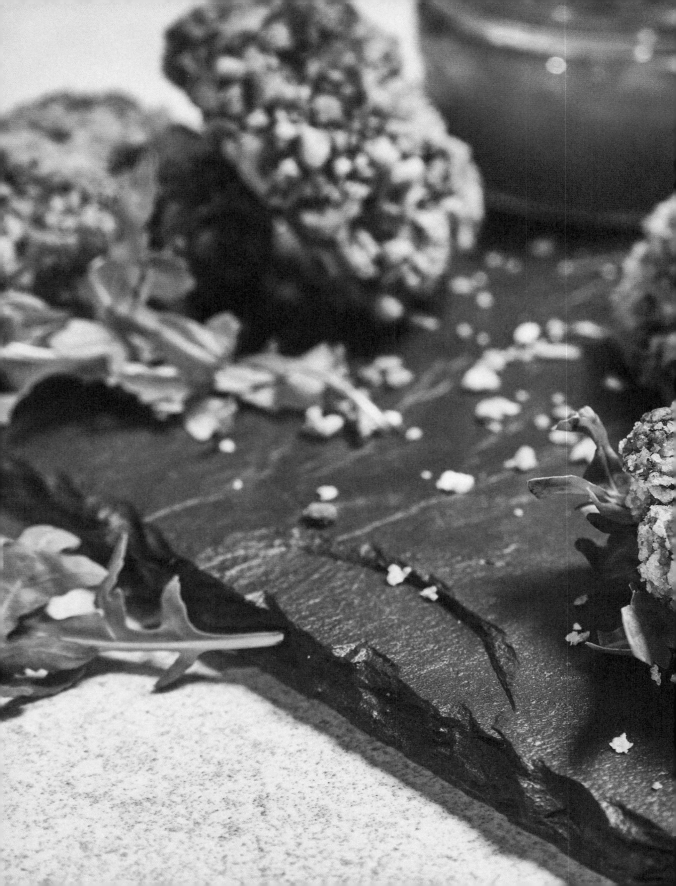

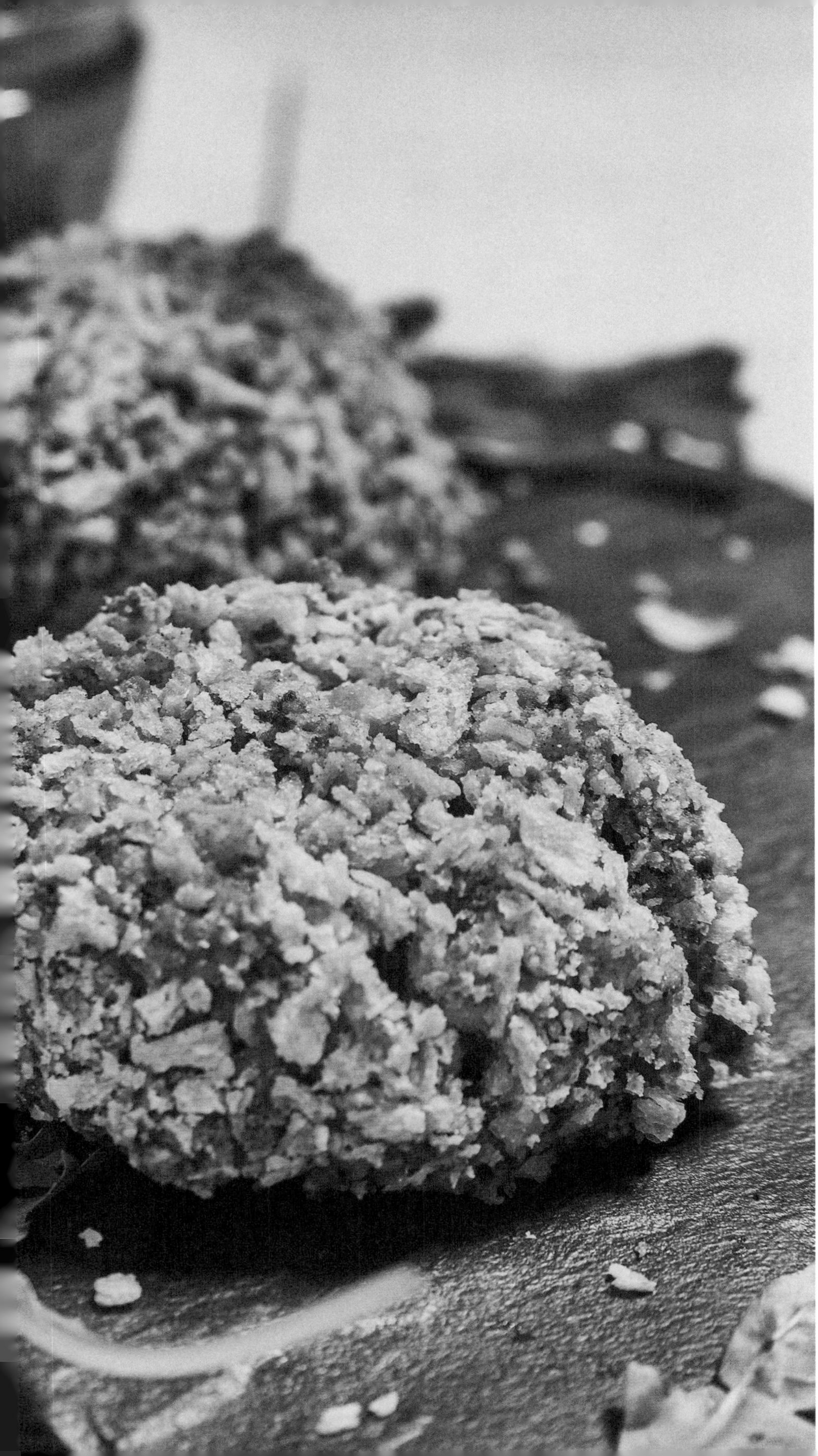

SIDES, DIPS & SAUCES

SIDES

DIPS

SAUCES

SIDES, DIPS & SAUCES

PESTO POTATOES

Serves 2

I love serving these potatoes with the Teriyaki, lemon and sesame greens as sides to a Sunday dinner feast – a Sunday dinner of dreams.

Ingredients

4 tbsp pesto (page 128)
200g white potatoes
200g sweet potatoes
2 tbsp olive oil
salt and black pepper to taste

1. Preheat the oven to 180°C and line a baking tray with baking paper.

2. Chop all the potatoes into cubes and add to a mixing bowl.

3. Stir in the olive oil, salt and pepper and mix well.

4. Spread the potatoes out evenly on the baking tray and cook in the oven for 20 minutes.

5. After 20 minutes, remove the tray from the oven and use a large spoon to carefully add the pesto to the potatoes, ensuring an even coverage.

6. Place the pesto potatoes back in the oven and cook for a further 10 minutes until the potatoes are cooked through.

SALT AND CHILLI CHIPS

Serves 2–4

Every time I go to a Chinese restaurant with my sister, the first thing she looks for on the menu is salt and chilli chips – so I make sure to always have this homemade version of her favourite dish ready for when she comes to visit.

Ingredients

4 large baking potatoes
1 green pepper, cut into slices
1 red pepper, cut into slices
2 tbsp soy sauce
1 white onion, cut into long pieces
1 tsp chilli flakes
1 tbsp olive oil
salt and pepper to taste

1. Preheat the oven to 180°C and line a baking tray with baking paper.

2. Cut the potatoes into wedges and add to a large mixing bowl with the onions and peppers.

3. Mix the olive oil, salt and pepper, soy sauce and chilli flakes together in a jug.

4. Pour the oil mix into a bowl and, using your hands, coat the potatoes, onion and pepper with it.

5. Spread the potatoes, onion and pepper evenly on the lined baking tray and bake in the oven for 30 to 40 minutes until the potatoes are cooked through.

6. These chips are delicious served as they are or as a side. I love them with Sesame orange seitan (page 80).

SIDES, DIPS & SAUCES

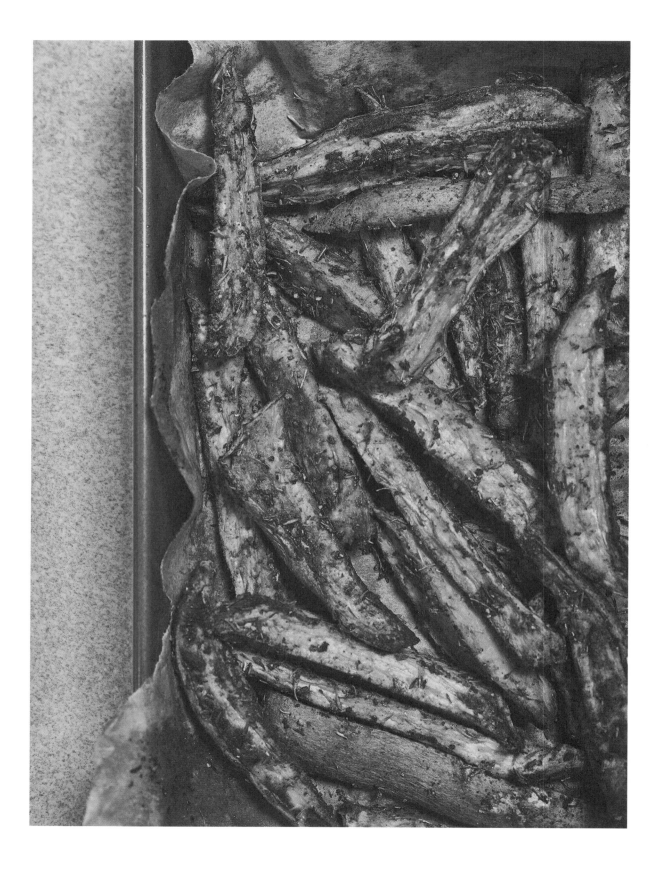

BAKED SWEET POTATO WEDGES WITH THYME

Serves 2–4

Nothing beats sweet potato wedges – any time I see them on a restaurant menu, or if I'm wanting a hearty side dish, I have to order them. These homemade wedges are super easy to make and can be added to a whole range of dishes – from nourish bowls to burgers!

Ingredients

4 large sweet potatoes
2 tbsp thyme
2 tbsp rosemary
1 tbsp paprika
1 tbsp olive oil
salt and pepper to taste

1. Preheat the oven to 180°C and line a baking tray with baking paper.

2. Cut the sweet potato into thick wedges and place in a large mixing bowl.

3. Mix together the olive oil, salt and pepper, paprika, rosemary and thyme in a jug.

4. Pour the oil mix into the bowl and, using your hands, coat the wedges with it.

5. Transfer the wedges to the baking tray and bake in the oven for 30 to 40 minutes until the potatoes are soft and cooked through.

6. Serve with a burger, in a nourish bowl, or just with your favourite condiments.

GARLIC AND BALSAMIC BRUSSELS SPROUTS

Serves 1–2

Brussels sprouts are, in my humble opinion, the best vegetable ever. However, I know they are like Marmite: you either love or hate them. This dish spices them up a little – so perhaps the Brussels sprout haters out there will be able to give them a second try!

Ingredients

200g Brussels sprouts
4 garlic cloves, minced
2 tbsp balsamic vinegar
1 tbsp olive oil
salt and pepper to taste

1. Preheat the oven to 180°C and line a baking tray with baking paper.

2. Peel and half the Brussels sprouts and add to a large mixing bowl.

3. Mix together the olive oil, garlic, balsamic vinegar, salt and pepper in a jug.

4. Pour the oil mix into the bowl and, using your hands, coat the sprouts with it.

5. Add the coated sprouts to the baking tray and cook in the oven for 15 to 20 minutes until crispy.

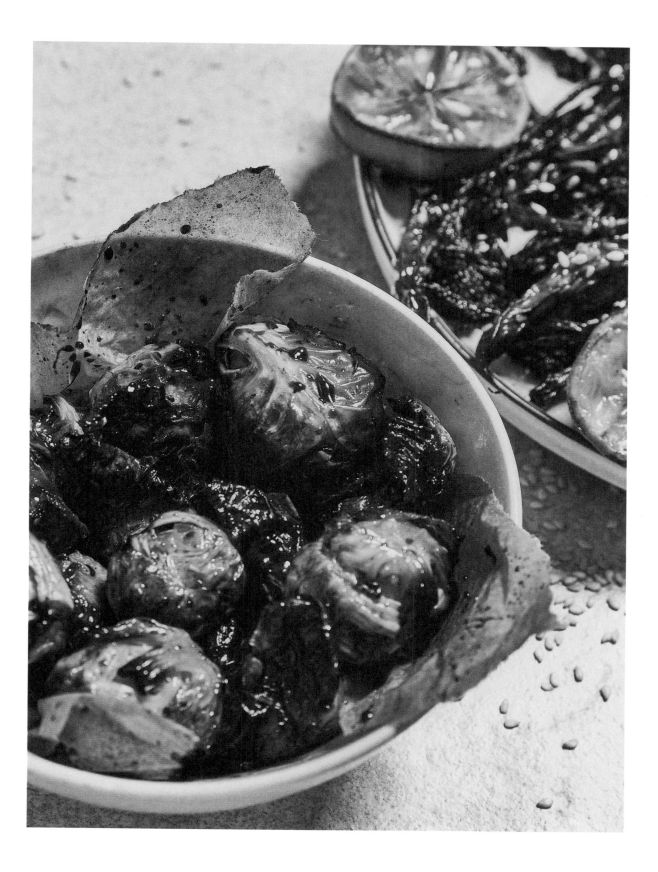

SPANISH BEANS AND SPINACH

Serves 2–4

Think ratatouille – but better. The base of rich tomato sauce mixed with beans and spinach makes the perfect accompaniment to any meal, or you can double the recipe and have it as a main.

Ingredients

2 tins chopped tomatoes
2 cans butter beans, drained and rinsed
2 large handfuls of spinach
1 tbsp olive oil
1 onion, diced
2 garlic cloves, minced
2 bay leaves
1 tsp smoked paprika
salt and black pepper to taste

1. First heat the olive oil in a preheated saucepan, then stir in the onion and garlic and sauté over a medium heat for a few minutes until the onion and garlic start to soften.

2. Add the smoked paprika and bay leaves and stir for another 1 to 2 minutes.

3. Stir in the chopped tomatoes, beans, spinach, salt and pepper, bring to the boil then turn down the heat and leave to simmer for 15 to 20 minutes.

4. Serve topped with an extra crack of black pepper.

SIDES, DIPS & SAUCES

BUFFALO TOFU SKEWERS

Makes 6

Summer is unreliable in Scotland, so I always try to pretend it's sunny by having BBQ-friendly foods that can be cooked in the kitchen while sheltering from the rain. These skewers are easy to make, and the vegetables can be switched out and replaced by whatever you have to hand.

Ingredients

1 block tofu
200g mushrooms
1 red pepper, chopped
1 yellow pepper, chopped
1 red onion, chopped
1 courgette, chopped
150g buffalo hot sauce
salt and pepper to taste

1. Preheat the oven to 180ºC and line a baking tray with baking paper.

2. Drain and remove the excess water from the tofu and cut into cubes.

3. In a bowl, coat the tofu in the buffalo hot sauce, add the salt and black pepper then spread it all out evenly on the lined baking tray.

4. Add the tofu to the skewers and bake in the oven for 10 minutes before removing and adding the chopped vegetables to the skewers.

5. Cook for another 10 to 15 minutes until the vegetables have softened and the tofu is firm and crispy.

TERIYAKI, LEMON AND
SESAME GREENS

Serves 1–2

*I'm always trying to find interested ways of adding more greens into my diet.
This dish is so tasty and can accompany so many main meals. I love serving it for
Sunday dinner – particularly with the Scottish Cottage Pie (page 86).*

Ingredients

100g asparagus
100g green beans
100g tenderstem broccoli
2 tbsp teriyaki sauce
2 tbsp sesame seeds
1 tbsp olive oil
½ lemon, juiced

1. Preheat the oven to 180°C and line a baking tray with baking paper.

2. Add the asparagus, green beans and broccoli to a bowl and coat in the olive oil and teriyaki sauce.

3. Spread the vegetables evenly onto the lined baking tray and cook in the oven for 10 minutes.

4. After 10 minutes, remove the vegetables from the oven, sprinkle over the sesame seeds and lemon juice and return to the oven for a further 5 minutes to finish cooking.

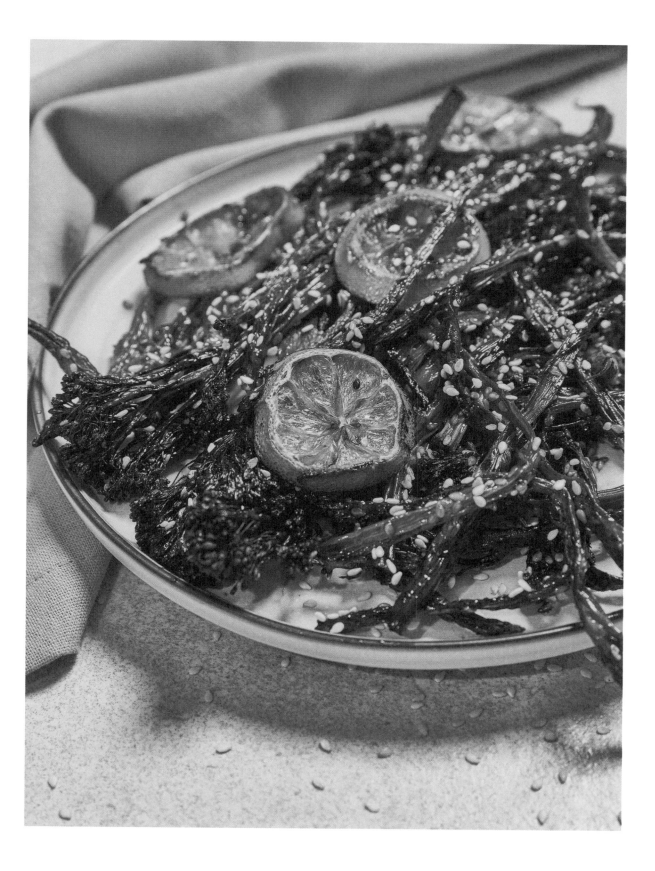

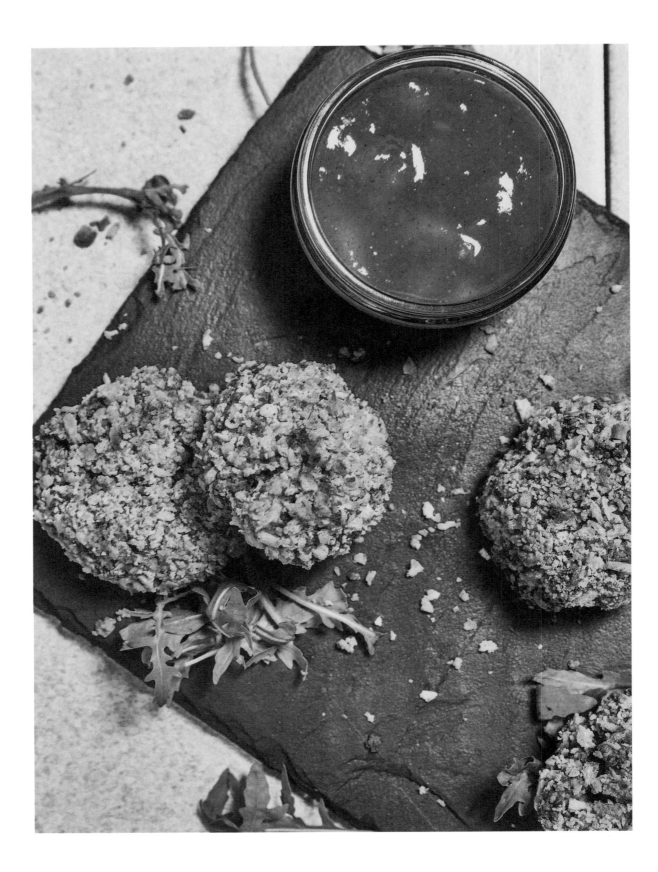

HAGGIS BON BONS WITH MANGO CHUTNEY

Makes 12–15

It might be a tad embarrassing to admit that, as a Scot, I have never actually tried (meat) haggis. However, now I'm vegan, I'm very happy I avoided it and can enjoy this delicious vegan option! This version is nutty and full of flavour and when combined with the dipping sauce is a showstopper, especially if you're looking to impress guests with your cooking skills.

Ingredients

500ml vegan stock
175g brown rice, cooked
100g Panko breadcrumbs
50g plain flour
100g green lentils, drained and rinsed
100g mushrooms
75g cashews
1 large carrot
1 large onion
4 tbsp olive oil
1 clove garlic
1 tbsp thyme
1 tbsp dark miso paste
½ tsp ground nutmeg

To serve

handful of rocket
4 tbsp mango chutney

1. Preheat the oven to 180°C.

2. In a food processor, combine the rice, onion, garlic, carrot, mushrooms and cashews until a chunky mixture forms – do not over-mix as you want a 'bite' to it.

3. Heat half of the olive oil in a pan and add in the vegetable mix. Cook until the vegetables starts to soften.

4. Stir in the thyme, miso paste, lentils and stock.

5. Bring to the boil, then reduce the heat and leave to simmer until the mixture has soaked up most of the moisture. If the mixture is still very liquid, add some cornstarch to thicken.

6. Using your hands, form the mix into 12 to 15 balls of haggis and set on a lined baking tray.

7. Take 3 separate bowls. Add the plain flour to one, the rest of the olive oil to the second, and the breadcrumbs to the third.

8. Coat each haggis ball in flour, then oil, then coat in breadcrumbs and return to the baking tray.

9. Bake in the oven for 40 minutes or until the breadcrumbs are golden and the ball is holding together well.

10. Serve on a bed of rocket with mango chutney for dipping.

HUMMUS

Serves 2–4

This simple recipe is one I make time and time again – and once you've made your own hummus, you'll never want to go back to shop-bought! Hummus is a staple part of the vegan diet and I love adding it to nourish bowls and burgers, or just as a snack with carrots and cucumber sticks.

Ingredients

1 tin chickpeas, drained and rinsed
2 tbsp tahini
2 garlic cloves
2 tbsp olive oil
½ lemon, juiced
3 tbsp water
pinch of salt

1. Add all of the ingredients to a blender or food processor and blend until smooth.

2. Serve immediately – or your hummus can be stored in an airtight container in the fridge for up to 3 days.

CHUNKY GUACAMOLE

Serves 2–4

Guacamole hardly needs an introduction. Creamy, rich and totally delicious, I love adding it to my nourish bowls, loading it on tortilla chips or just spreading it on toast for a quick and healthy snack. It's also a great crowd pleaser and I often double the recipe if I'm serving it – just to make sure everyone gets their fair share!

Ingredients

2 avocados, stones removed and roughly sliced
½ red onion, diced
2 garlic cloves, minced
handful of fresh coriander
1 fresh chilli, finely chopped
1 lime, juiced
salt and black pepper to taste

1. Add all of the ingredients to a food processor and pulse until the desired consistency is reached. I like to keep it a little chunky but for a smoother texture, blend it for a little longer. Don't have a food processor? You can use a hand whisk or a fork to simply mash all the ingredients together.

2. Serve immediately – or your guacamole can be stored in an airtight container in the fridge for up to 3 days.

SIDES, DIPS & SAUCES

HOMEMADE SALSA – 3 WAYS

Serves 2–4

Salsa. The sassiest of sauces. Three ways.

1. Mild

1 tin chopped tomatoes
2 garlic cloves, minced
½ cucumber, chopped into cubes
½ red onion, diced
½ tbsp paprika
handful of fresh coriander, roughly chopped
1 lime, juiced
salt and pepper to taste

2. Jalapeño

1 tin chopped tomatoes
½ red onion, diced
1 large jalapeño pepper, finely chopped
2 garlic cloves, minced
½ tbsp paprika
1 lime, juiced
1 tsp chilli powder
handful of fresh coriander, roughly chopped
salt and pepper to taste

3. Mango

4 large tomatoes, chopped
1 mango, stone removed and sliced
1 red pepper, chopped into cubes
½ red onion, diced
½ cucumber, chopped into cubes
1 lime, juiced
handful of fresh coriander
salt and pepper to taste

1. For all 3 salsas, add all your ingredients to a food processor and pulse until combined but still chunky.

2. Serve immediately – or your salsa can be stored in an airtight container in the fridge for up to 3 days.

GARLIC AND TOMATO PASTA SAUCE

Serves 2–4

Pasta is a go-to meal in many households. This garlic and tomato sauce is super easy to make and will elevate any basic pasta dish. Make sure you leave it to simmer so the delicious flavours of the garlic and spices can infuse into the tomatoes.

Ingredients

3 tbsp tomato paste
2 tins chopped tomatoes
½ white onion, diced
3 garlic cloves, minced
1 tbsp olive oil
1 tbsp smoked paprika
1 tsp chilli powder
½ tbsp dried basil
½ tbsp dried oregano
salt and black pepper

1. Heat the oil in a preheated, non-stick pan then add the onion and garlic. Sauté until they start to soften.

2. Stir in the tomato paste, paprika, chilli powder, salt, pepper, basil and oregano.

3. Then add the chopped tomatoes. Now bring to the boil before turning down the heat and allowing to simmer for at least 30 minutes.

TAHINI, LEMON AND CHILLI SALAD DRESSING

Serves 2–4

This rich, creamy dressing is perfect for salads or paired with falafel.

Ingredients

3 tbsp tahini
2 tbsp maple syrup
2 tbsp water
1 tbsp chilli flakes
½ lemon, juiced
salt and black pepper

1. Combine all the ingredients in a bowl and stir until smooth.

EASY PEASY PESTO

Serves 2–4

You might think pesto is complicated to make – but it's really quite simple! I love adding this to pasta dishes and drizzling over nourish bowls or roast veggies to add an extra kick of flavour.

Ingredients

150ml olive oil
50g pine nuts
50g cashew nuts OR vegan parmesan
2 garlic cloves, minced
large bunch of fresh basil

1. Blend all of the ingredients in a food processor or blender until smooth.

2. Enjoy immediately – or store in an airtight container in the fridge for up to 3 days.

AVOCADO AND HERB SALAD DRESSING

Serves 2–4

Coat your salad with this creamy avocado dressing for a fresh summer flavour.

Ingredients

1 avocado
4 tbsp olive oil
2 garlic cloves
1 lime, juiced
1 handful of fresh coriander
black pepper to taste

1. Add all of your ingredients to a food processor or blender and pulse until smooth.

SIDES, DIPS & SAUCES

CHIA STRAWBERRY JAM

Makes 1 small jar

Jam feels so British – I always associate it with afternoon tea with scones and empire biscuits or in a Victoria sponge cake. This version of the traditional preserve has a healthy twist, using chia seeds for added nutrients and crunch. I love adding it to pancakes, French toast or waffles as an extra sweet topping.

Ingredients

400g strawberries
2 tbsp chia seeds
2 tbsp maple syrup
½ lemon, juiced

1. Add all of the ingredients to a food processor or blender and blend until smooth. The chia seeds will thicken the mixture and add a gel-like consistency.

2. Enjoy immediately – or store in an airtight container in the fridge for 3 days.

CHOCOLATE FUDGE SAUCE

Serves 2

I am a chocoholic and this recipe is deliciously indulgent and proves that you don't need to give up chocolate to enjoy a plant-based lifestyle.

Ingredients

2 tbsp coconut oil
2 tbsp maple syrup
2 tbsp cacao powder, or more depending on desired consistency. The more powder, the thicker the sauce

1. Melt the coconut oil in a pan or using the microwave. Once melted add to a bowl with the maple syrup and cacao.

2. Whisk until a smooth sauce is formed – this can take a few minutes.

3. Enjoy immediately – or store in an airtight container in the fridge and add to pancakes, waffles or as an ice cream topping.

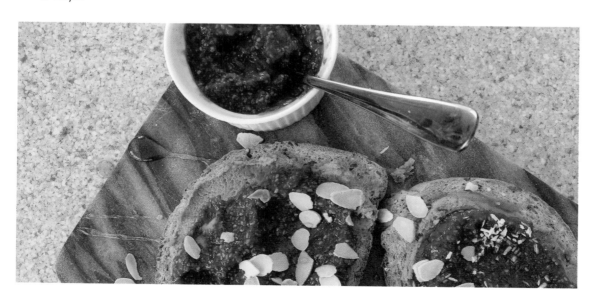

SIDES, DIPS & SAUCES

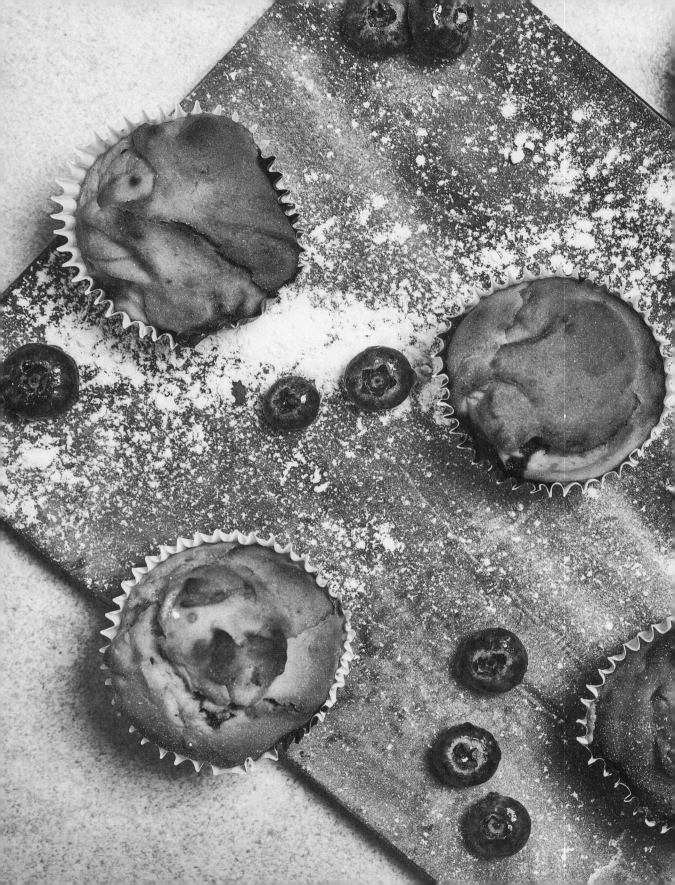

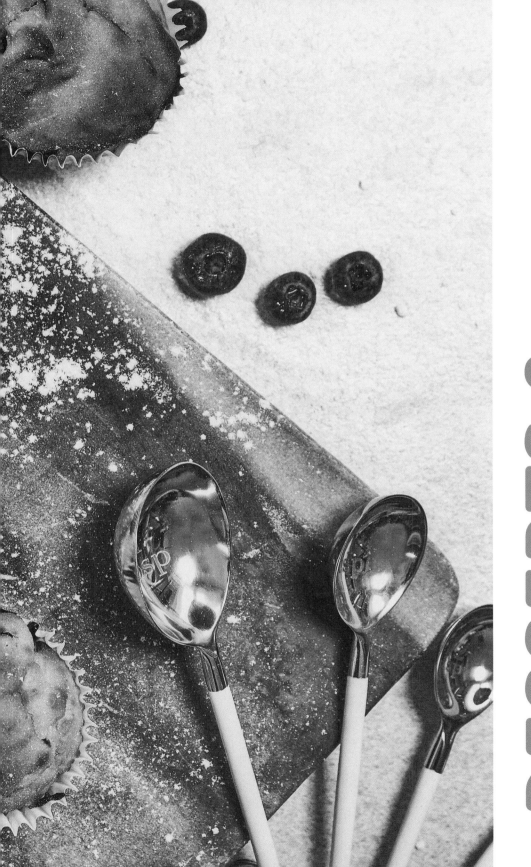

DESSERTS &
SWEET SNACKS

INSTANT MUG CAKE
– 3 WAYS

PROTEIN BALLS – 4 WAYS

PROTEIN BARS – 2 WAYS

DESSERTS & SWEET SNACKS

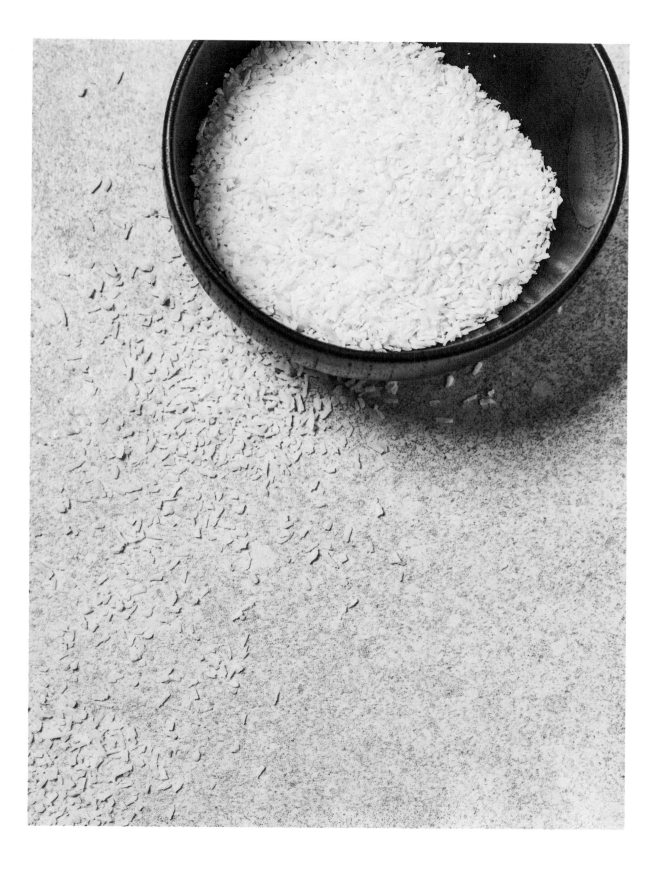

INSTANT MUG CAKE – 3 WAYS

Each recipe makes 1 cake

Sometimes all you really want is cake. But making a whole cake, just for yourself, can be a struggle. Enter the mug cake! Easy and ready in less than five minutes, it's perfect for those evenings when you need comfort food – a hug in a mug.

1. CHOCOLATE

Ingredients

2 tbsp plain flour
2 tbsp cocoa powder
3 tbsp non-dairy milk
2 tbsp coconut sugar
1 tbsp melted coconut oil
½ tsp vanilla extract
¼ tsp baking powder.
pinch of salt

2. RASPBERRY AND VANILLA

Ingredients

3 tbsp plain flour
3 tbsp non-dairy milk
2 tbsp coconut sugar
1 tbsp vanilla protein powder or substitute with
   1 tbsp flour
1 tbsp melted coconut oil
½ tsp vanilla extract
¼ tsp baking powder.
pinch of salt
handful of raspberries

1. For both mug cakes, start by mixing together the dry ingredients before adding in the wet.

2. Pour the mixture into a microwave-friendly mug.

3. Cook for 60 seconds in a high-powered microwave. Insert a thin-bladed knife into the centre of the cake. If it comes out clean the cake is ready; if not, microwave the cake for another 20 seconds until cooked.

3. CINNAMON ROLL

Ingredients

3 tbsp plain flour
3 tbsp non-dairy milk
2 tbsp coconut sugar
1 tbsp vanilla protein powder or
   substitute with 1 tbsp flour
1 tbsp melted coconut oil
½ tsp cinnamon
¼ tsp baking powder
pinch of salt

For the sauce

1-2 tbsp almond milk
60-100g icing sugar

1. Start by mixing together the dry ingredients before adding in the wet.

2. Pour the mixture into a microwave-friendly mug.

3. Cook for 60 seconds in a high-powered microwave. Insert a thin-bladed knife into the centre of the cake. If it comes out clean the cake is ready; if not, microwave the cake for another 20 seconds until cooked.

4. Mix together the powdered sugar with the almond milk to create a sauce and pour over the cake to serve.

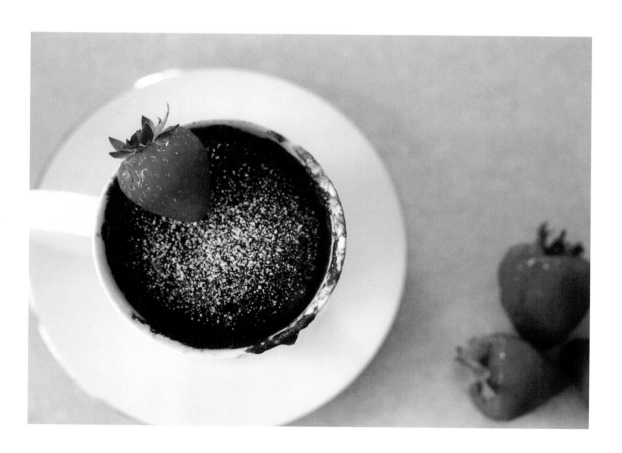

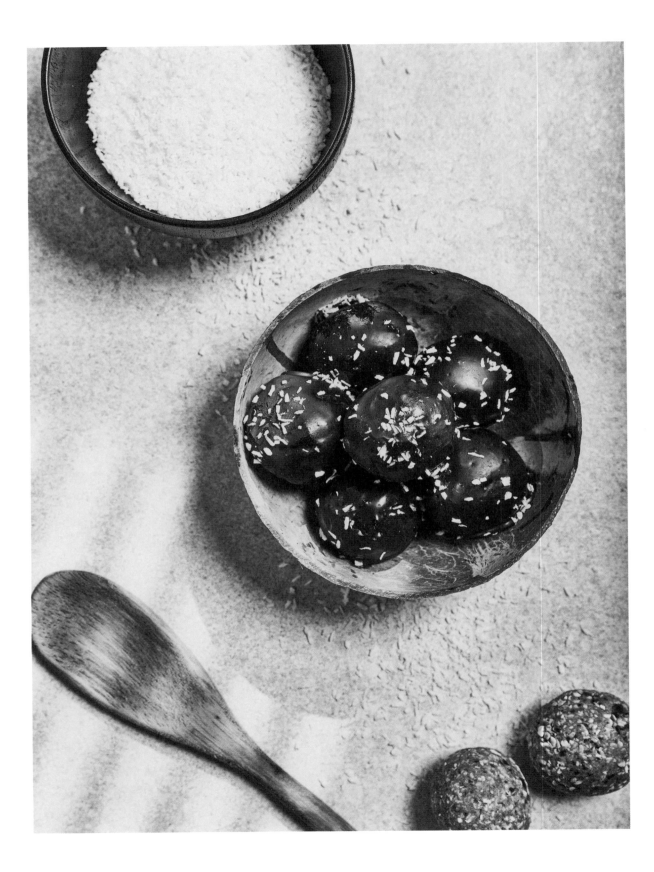

PROTEIN BALLS
- 4 WAYS

Each recipe makes 8–10 balls

I make these protein balls at least once a week. They're super easy to make and store in the fridge – the perfect snack to grab on-the-go or if you need an extra boost of energy before your workout!

1. VANILLA AND COCONUT

Ingredients

150g medjool dates, pitted
100g vegan-friendly chocolate
120g oats
60g vanilla protein powder
40g desiccated coconut

2. RASPBERRY AND DARK CHOCOLATE

Ingredients

150g medjool dates, pitted
100g vegan-friendly chocolate
50g freeze-dried raspberries
120g oats
60g vanilla protein powder
40g desiccated coconut

1. In a blender or food processor, combine the dates, oats, protein and coconut until a stiff mixture forms – be careful to avoid over-blending.

2. If you are making the raspberry balls, blend half of the freeze-dried raspberries into the mixture.

3. Roll the mix into balls and store in the fridge.

4. Melt the vegan chocolate and then carefully coat each ball with it and place back in the fridge to set.

5. If you are making the raspberry balls, scatter the other half of freeze-dried raspberries over the top of the chocolate-covered balls before placing them back in the fridge to set.

3. COOKIE DOUGH

Ingredients

1 x 400g tin chickpeas, drained and rinsed
100g vegan chocolate
40g vanilla protein powder
3 tbsp cashew nut butter
4 tbsp maple syrup
4 tbsp coconut flour

4. PEANUT BUTTER

Ingredients

1 x 400g tin chickpeas, drained and rinsed
100g vegan chocolate
40g vanilla protein powder
3 tbsp peanut nut butter
4 tbsp maple syrup
4 tbsp coconut flour

1. In a blender or food processor add the chickpeas, protein powder, nut butter, syrup and coconut flour until smooth.

2. Roll the mix into balls and store in the fridge.

3. Melt the vegan chocolate and and carefully coat each ball with it. Then place back in the fridge to set.

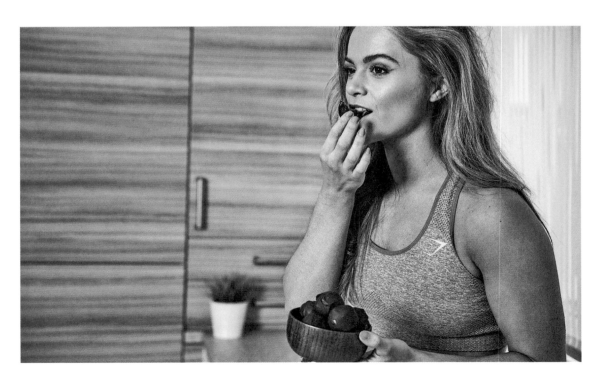

DESSERTS & SWEET SNACKS

PROTEIN BARS – 2 WAYS

Each recipe makes 8 bars

Protein bars are great snacks, but they can be expensive to buy and also full of questionable ingredients. These homemade bars are money-saving and healthy. You can store them in an airtight container for up to 5 days in the fridge.

1. PEANUT AND CHOCOLATE CHIP

Ingredients

150g dates, pitted
90g vanilla protein powder
240g brown rice puffed cereal
60g oats
60g desiccated coconut
60g peanut butter
4 tbsp maple syrup

Optional vegan chocolate

1. In a food processor or blender, pulse together the oats, coconut, half of the protein powder and dates to form a sticky base to the protein bar.

2. Line a baking tin with baking paper and spread and press the mixture flat over the base of the tin.

3. In a large mixing bowl, mix together the cereal, peanut butter, the rest of the protein powder and maple syrup. Then spread this on top of the base layer.

4. As an optional layer, melt the vegan chocolate in a pan or microwave and pour evenly over the bars.

5. Place the tin in the fridge for at least 2 hours until the layers have set.

6. Remove from the fridge and cut into 8 equal bars.

2. MINT CHOCOLATE CRISP

Ingredients

150g dates, pitted
90g vanilla protein powder
4 tbsp maple syrup
240g brown rice puffed cereal
60g oats
60g desiccated coconut
60g cashew butter
1 tsp mint extract

1. In a food processor or blender, pulse the oats, coconut, half of the protein powder and dates to form a sticky base to the protein bar.

2. Add to a baking tin lined with baking paper and press flat.

3. In a bowl combine the cereal, cashew butter, mint extract, the rest of the protein powder and maple syrup until well combined and spread out on top of the base layer and refrigerate until the layers have set together.

4. Remove from the fridge and cut into 8 equal bars.

5. Melt your favourite vegan chocolate and evenly coat the bars.

6. Return to the fridge to set.

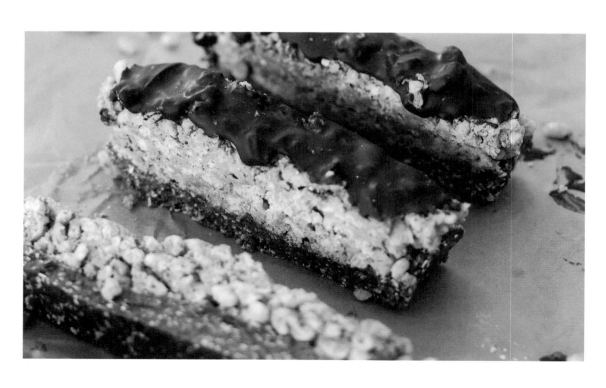

TRAIL MIX BARS

Makes 8

Trail mix bars – nuts and seeds squished together with dates and chocolate make for one of the most epic snacks of all time. Whether you're actually hiking a trail or just hanging out with friends, these bars are totally delicious.

Ingredients

200g fruit and nut mix of your choice,
  plus extra for topping
150g medjool dates, pitted
100g dried mango, cut into small chunks
  (plus extra for topping)
75g oats

For the ganache topping

4-6 tbsp raw cacao powder
2 tbsp coconut oil, melted
2 tbsp maple syrup

1. Start by blending the dates, oats and fruit and nut mix in a blender or food processor to form a sticky / crumbly mix, then stir in the mango chunks.

2. Transfer the mixture to a lined baking tin and press it evenly across the tin to form the base layer of the bars.

3. Place in the fridge to set for 10 to 15 minutes.

4. Mix together the ganache ingredients to form a thick, chocolatey sauce.

5. Remove the tray from the fridge and spread the ganache over the top of base layer, then sprinkle on the remainder of fruit, nut and mango over the ganache.

6. Place in the fridge for about 30 minutes until the ganache topping has set.

7. Slice into 8 squares. These bars will keep in an airtight container in the fridge for 3 to 5 days.

ALMOND AND SEA SALT
BLACK BEAN BROWNIES

Makes 10

*Brownies – with a healthy twist. Once a cheeky little snack, these are
protein-packed and full of nutrients, good for the body and soul.*

Ingredients

65g almond flour or ground almonds
20g coconut oil
1 x tin of black beans, drained and rinsed
150g coconut sugar
60ml almond milk
90g raw cacao powder
60g chocolate protein powder or
  substitute with 60g of flour
60g almond butter

Toppings

200g vegan dark chocolate
handful of almonds
1 tsp sea salt

1. Preheat the oven to 160°C and grease or line a rectangular baking tin with baking paper.

2. Blend the brownie ingredients together in a blender until a smooth batter is formed.

3. Pour the brownie mixture into the lined tin and cook in the oven for 60 minutes. Check the brownies are cooked by inserting a thin-bladed knife into the centre of the tin. If the knife comes out clean, they are ready.

4. While the brownies cool, melt the chocolate in a bowl over a pan of boiling water or microwave. Pour the melted chocolate over the brownies, then scatter over the almonds and sea salt.

5. Pop the tin in the fridge for at least an hour, overnight if possible, then remove and cut into squares.

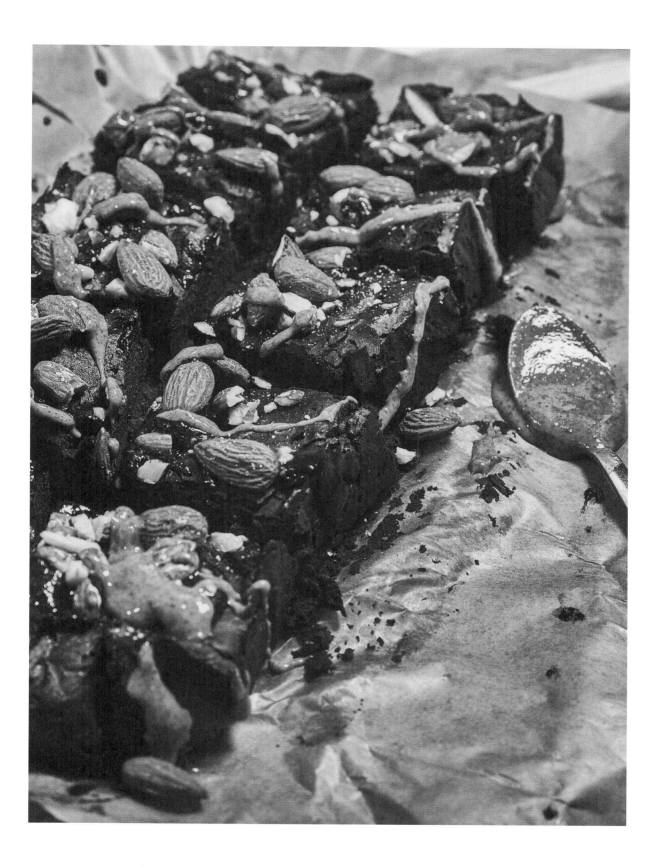

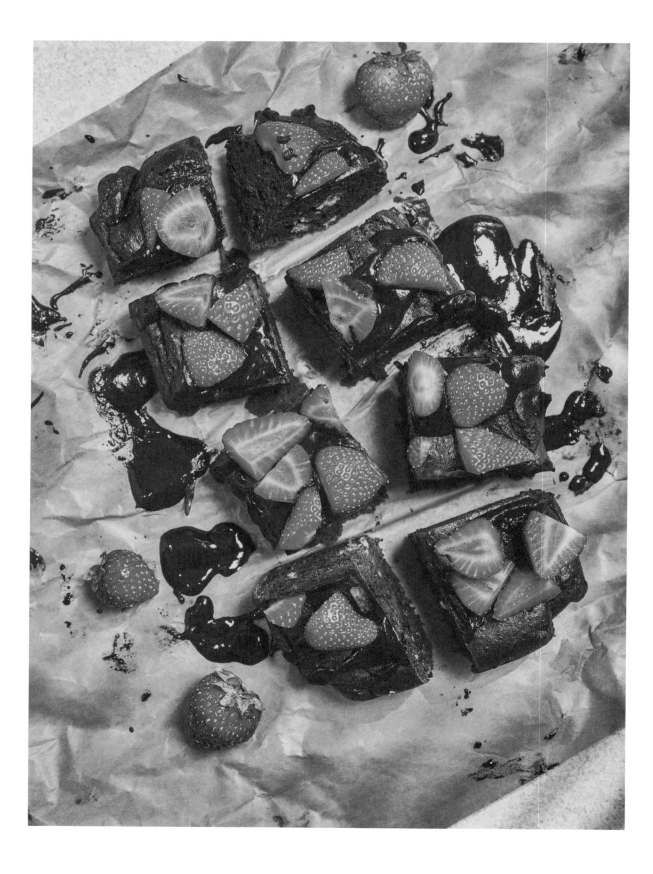

CHOCOLATE AND STRAWBERRY LOAF

Serves 8

I made this on Valentine's Day for my hubby, Marco, and it turned out to be quite a success!
But it doesn't have to be limited to Valentine's Day, I love making this on all special occasions.

Ingredients

230ml almond milk
1 tsp vinegar
120g plain flour
90g coconut sugar
60g mashed banana
40g cacao powder
½ tsp baking powder
¼ tsp salt

For the ganache

90g cacao powder
60ml melted coconut oil
60ml pure maple syrup
200g fresh strawberries (or any fresh
  berries of your choice)

1. Preheat the oven to 180°C and line a loaf tin with baking paper.

2. Mix together the almond milk, vinegar and mashed banana in a bowl.

3. In a separate bowl, combine the flour, cacao, baking powder, salt and coconut sugar.

4. Add the wet mixture to the dry and stir until fully combined to form the cake batter.

5. Pour the cake mixture into the lined tin and cook in the oven for 25 to 30 minutes or until a knife comes out clean from the centre.

6. While the cake cooks, melt together the ganache ingredients in a saucepan or in the microwave.

7. Remove the cake from the oven. Leave to cool for a few minutes in the tin and turn out onto a wire rack to cool fully.

8. Transfer the cake to a plate or cake stand before pouring over the ganache and topping with the strawberries.

9. Place in the fridge to set for at least an hour before serving.

CHOCOLATE CARAMEL SLICES

Makes 10

The good old caramel slice. Ah, we really do love you. Try out this healthy version of the classic caramel shortcake for a grab-and-go snack or a quick evening dessert throughout the week.

Ingredients

350g dates, pitted
100g vegan chocolate
100ml water
50g vanilla protein powder or substitute
    with 50g oats
2 tbsp almond butter
60g oats
60g desiccated coconut
1 tsp vanilla extract
sea salt to taste

1. Start by blending 150 grams of the dates, protein powder, oats and coconut in a blender or food processer to form a sticky, crumbly mix.

2. Transfer the mixture to a lined baking tin and press it evenly across the base of the tin to form the biscuit-like base layer of the caramel slices.

3. Place in the fridge to set while you make the caramel.

4. Use a blender or food processer to blend together the rest of the dates, vanilla extract, water and almond butter

5. Remove the baking tin from the fridge and spread the caramel over the biscuit-like base then place the tray in the freezer for 15 minutes.

6. While the caramel sets, melt the vegan chocolate either in a bowl over boiling water on the hob or in the microwave.

7. Remove the tray from the freezer and pour the melted chocolate over the caramel, then top with a sprinkle of sea salt.

8. Return to the fridge until the caramel slices are fully set.

9. Cut into 10 equal squares and serve with tea or coffee for a perfect afternoon pick-me-up.

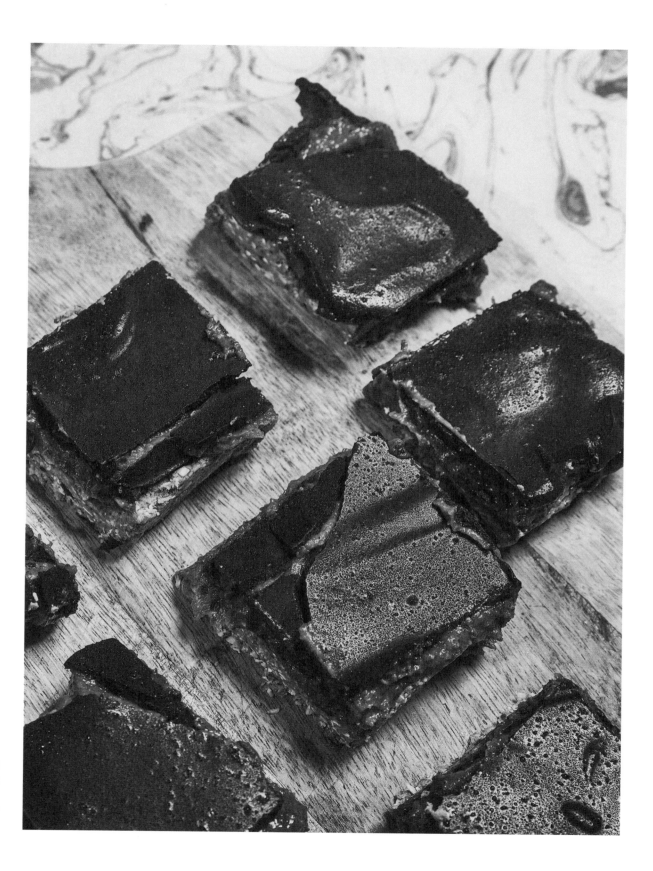

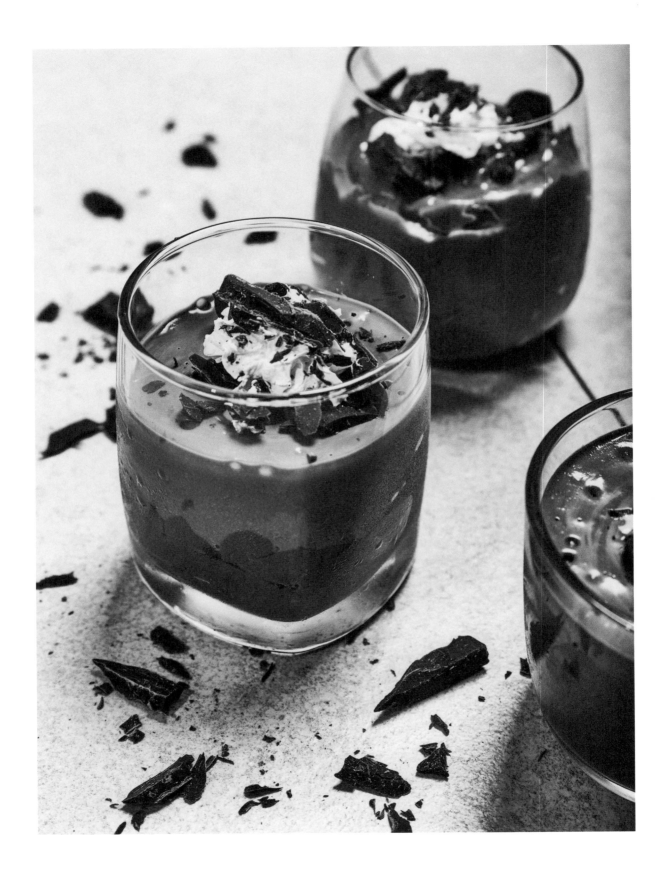

TOFU CHOCOLATE MOUSSE

Makes 3

I know, tofu and chocolate do not sound like a winning combination but, trust me, this mousse is utterly delicious. Served in cocktail glasses or ramekins, it's a perfect pudding for dinner parties.

Ingredients

300g silken tofu
100g vegan-friendly chocolate
80g maple syrup
1 tsp vanilla extract
pinch of sea salt

1. First melt the chocolate in a bowl over a pan of boiling water or in the microwave.

2. Drain and remove excess moisture from the tofu.

3. Add the tofu, maple syrup, vanilla and salt to a food processor and combine until smooth.

4. Then add in the melted chocolate and pulse until well combined.

5. Pour the mixture into ramekin-style dishes, filling up around a quarter of the dish and place in the fridge to set.

6. To serve, top with vegan whipped cream and chocolate – optional!

CHOCOLATE CHIP OAT COOKIES

Makes 6

The recipe for these cookies was created entirely by accident when my hungry sister wanted a pre-dinner snack. As you'll see, they're very easy to make, so they're perfect to turn to next time you have a hunger-related emergency!

Ingredients

2 ripe bananas
2 tbsp chocolate chips
120g oats
40g vanilla protein powder
1 tbsp cashew nut butter

1. Preheat the oven to 180°C and line a baking tray with baking paper.

2. Mash the bananas in a bowl and then stir in all of the other ingredients to make a dough.

3. Using your hands, make 6 cookies and place them evenly on the lined baking tray.

4. Cook in the oven for 15 to 18 minutes until they are golden on the outside but still soft in the middle.

5. Remove and allow to cool on a wire rack before serving.

DESSERTS & SWEET SNACKS

149

BANANA BREAD

Serves 8–10

This banana bread recipe is super easy to make and is perfect for an afternoon snack or to have in your kitchen when friends come over. It's great to bake on a Sunday and store in a tub in the fridge to enjoy as a snack throughout the week.

Ingredients

2 very ripe bananas
190g oat flour
100g coconut sugar
60g vanilla protein powder or substitute
    with 60g oat flour
40g coconut oil
1 tsp baking soda
½ tsp baking powder
1 tsp vanilla extract
1 tsp apple cider vinegar
½ tsp salt
100ml water

For the icing

4 tbsp icing sugar
1 tbsp vanilla protein
1 tbsp almond milk

If you prefer your banana bread less sweet, you can skip the icing – I love toasting a couple of slices with nut butter and my homemade chia jam.

1. Preheat the oven to 180°C.

2. In a large mixing bowl, stir together the flour, protein powder, baking powder, baking soda, salt and coconut sugar.

3. In a separate bowl, mash the bananas and add the vanilla extract, vinegar and water. Stir to make a smooth mixture.

4. Combine the dry and wet mixtures to form the cake batter. Pour into a greased, lined loaf tin and cook for 25 to 30 minutes.

5. Make the icing while the banana bread cooks. In a large mixing bowl, stir together the icing sugar, almond milk and protein so the mixture is smooth but not too runny. Add more or less milk accordingly.

6. To check if your banana bread is cooked, do the 'knife test'. Insert a thin-bladed knife into the centre of the loaf. If the knife comes out clean, the bread is ready. Remove the cooked loaf from the oven then leave to cool in the tin for 10 minutes before gently removing from the tin.

7. Allow to cool fully on a wire rack before adding the icing.

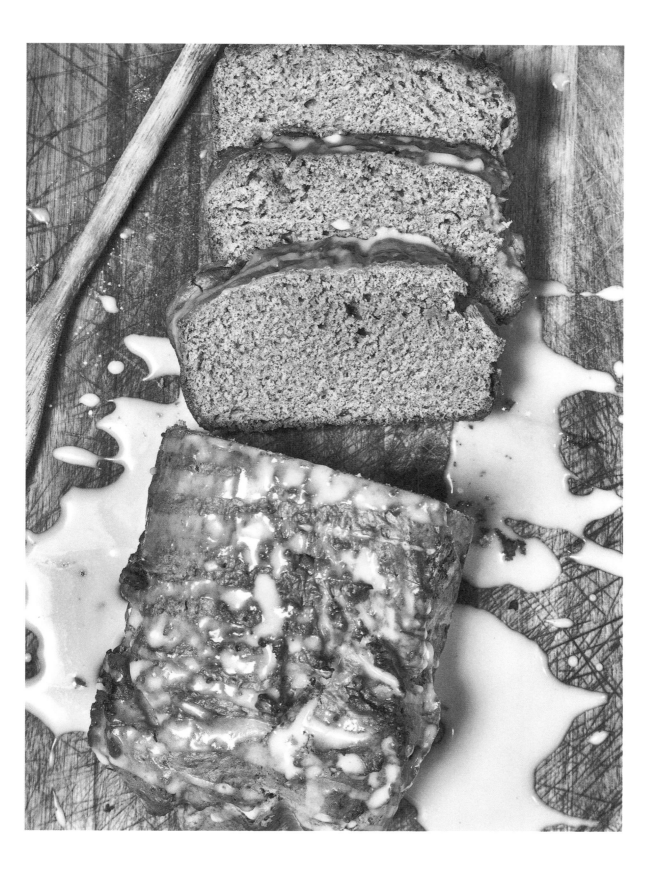

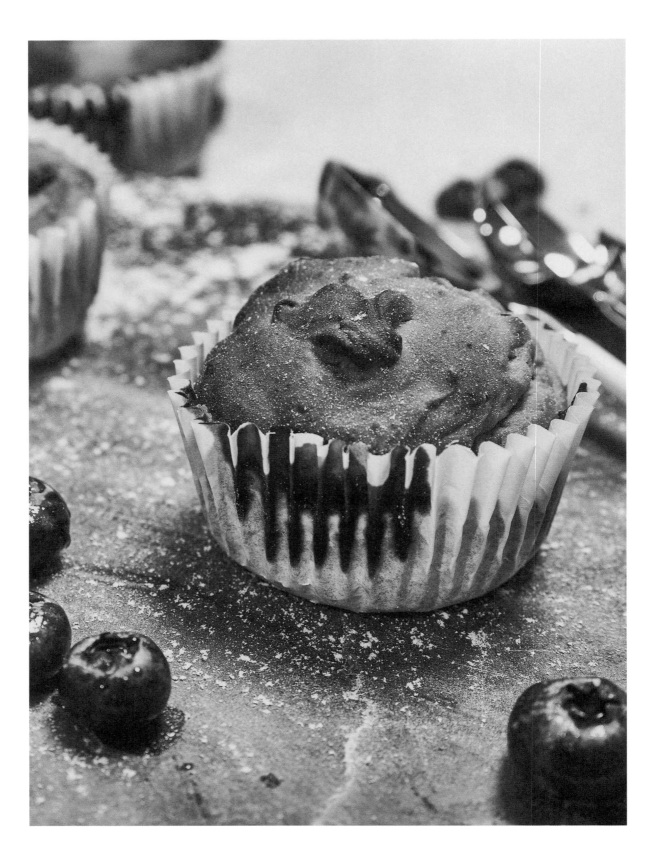

OAT AND BLUEBERRY MUFFINS

Makes 12

These muffins are the perfect snack when you need something sweet but healthy – a good option to reach for instead of the not-so-healthy chocolate or bag of salty, fried food that will have you feeling like a slug. I do not want you to feel like a slug, I want you to feel like a butterfly – and these muffins are butterfly-material!

Ingredients

225g oat flour, you can make this by
   blending oats to a fine powder
150ml almond milk
130ml maple syrup
75g vanilla protein powder or substitute
   with 75g of flour
120g blueberries
60g vegan yogurt (plain)
1 tbsp corn starch
1 tsp vanilla
1 tsp cider vinegar
1 lemon, juiced

1. Preheat the oven to 180°C and place 12 muffin cases into a muffin tray.

2. Start by mixing together the oat flour, cornstarch and protein powder.

3. Add this mixture to a bowl and slowly stir in the rest of the ingredients, leaving out the blueberries.

4. Once the wet and dry ingredients have formed a batter, add the blueberries.

5. Divide the mixture evenly into the muffin cases and bake in the oven for 20 minutes.

6. Once cooked, remove from the oven and transfer the muffins onto a wire rack. Allow to cool for 10 to 15 minutes before serving.

7. The muffins can be stored in an airtight container and eaten within a few days.

DESSERTS & SWEET SNACKS

PEANUT BUTTER CUPS

Makes 12

Another recipe inspired by my travels in America. This healthier take on the classic peanut butter cup includes an optional spoon of protein powder for a great post-workout boost.

Ingredients

100g vegan-friendly chocolate
2 tbsp peanut butter
1 tbsp maple syrup
1 tbsp coconut oil
1 tbsp vanilla protein powder, optional

1. To begin, place cupcake cases into a muffin baking tray.

2. Melt together the peanut butter, syrup, oil and protein powder in a large saucepan over a medium heat.

3. Melt your vegan chocolate in a separate pan.

4. Add a tablespoon of the melted chocolate to each cupcake case and then pop the tray in the fridge until the chocolate sets.

5. Remove the tray and add a layer of the peanut butter mix to each cupcake case before returning to fridge.

6. As you wait for the peanut butter mix to set, check if your melted chocolate is still melted – if not, reheat so it returns to liquid form.

7. Remove the peanut butter cups from the fridge and add a final layer of the melted chocolate. Then return to the fridge to set for one last time.

8. Enjoy immediately or store in an airtight container in the fridge for up to 3 days.

HOT CHOCOLATE PROTEIN SHAKE

Serves 1

Hot chocolate has got to be one of the most comforting things on the planet. Whether it is winter or summer, it's a drink I always turn to. This recipe uses almond milk, but you could substitute with any non-dairy milk of your choice.

Ingredients

2 tbsp raw cacao powder
380ml almond milk
1 tbsp chocolate protein powder
1 tsp vanilla extract
1 tbsp maple syrup

1. Combine all of the ingredients in a saucepan over a medium heat and whisk until well combined.

2. Serve hot. Vegan marshmallows and cream are optional but highly recommended!

THE ULTIMATE PEANUT BUTTER MILKSHAKE

Serves 1

A few small adjustments to a regular breakfast smoothie created this epic dessert milkshake – one of my favourite post-dinner snacks!

Ingredients

20g vanilla protein powder, optional
2 frozen bananas
250ml almond milk
1 tbsp peanut butter
1 tsp vanilla extract
handful vegan chocolate chips
vegan whipped cream

1. In a blender, combine the bananas, peanut butter, milk, protein powder and vanilla extract.

2. Stir in the chocolate chips, then pulse the blender once or twice to break up the chips.

3. Pour the milkshake into a sundae or milkshake glass and serve with a dollop of vegan whipped cream.

4. Drink up!

DESSERTS & SWEET SNACKS

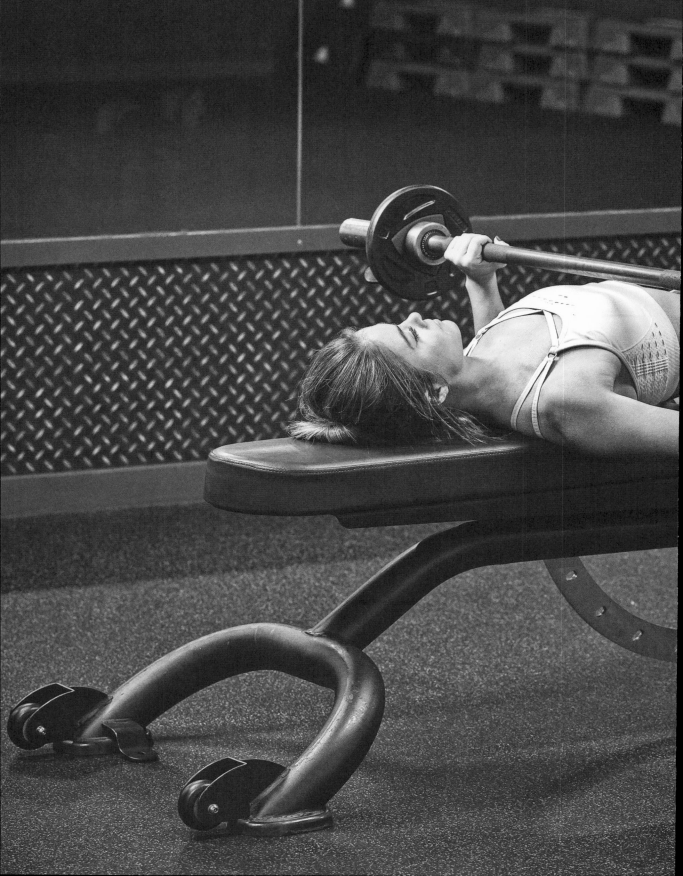

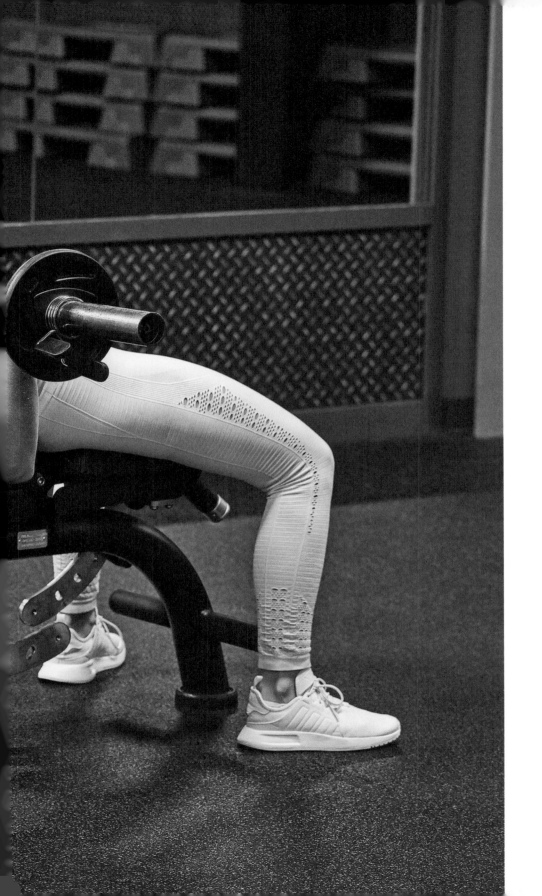

WORKOUTS

'I LOVE training and I love it because it is a never-ending journey: there is no final destination that you will reach and finally be "happy". You have to enjoy each workout and each healthy meal and know you are doing good for your body, not punishing it.

Don't work out to counteract what you have eaten; use what you have eaten to fuel your workout. That is the mindset I would love you to have. Learn to push your body to see what it can achieve; every small achievement is an achievement.'

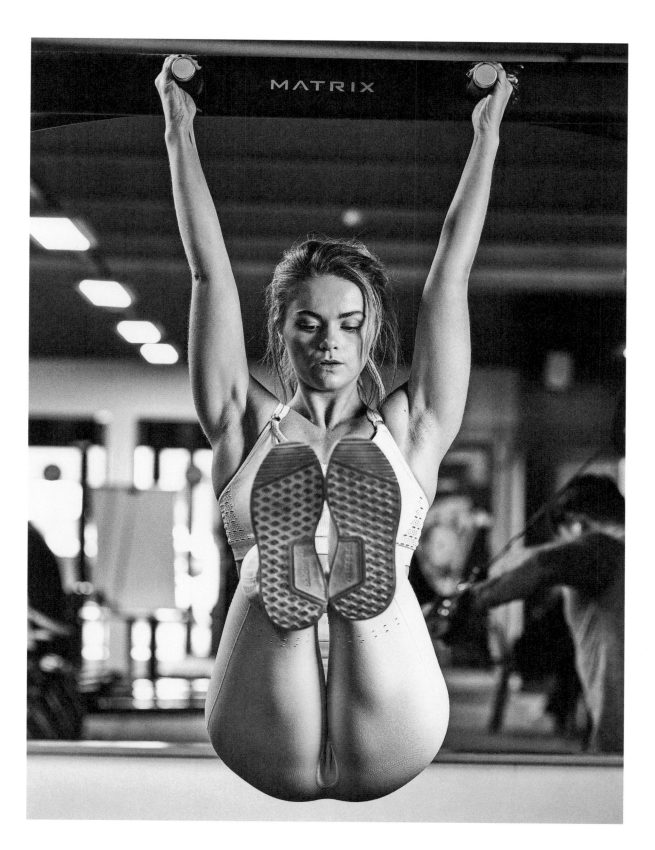

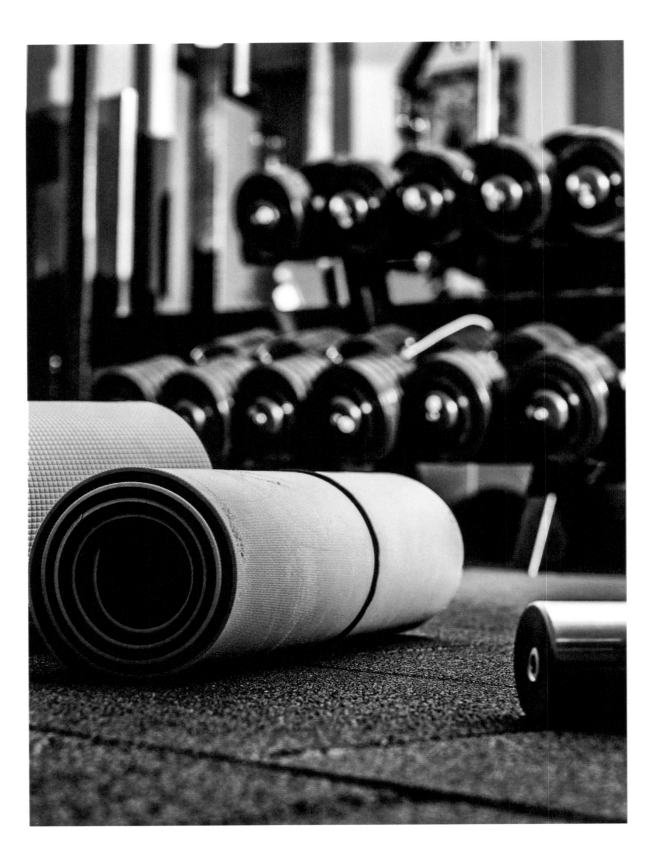

WHY EXERCISE?

Exercise is an integral part of living a healthy lifestyle. Many people view exercise as a way to look better, either to lose weight or change their body shape in some way. There is absolutely nothing wrong with that, but it is important to have reasons to exercise other than just the aesthetic benefits. If you only view exercise as a way to lose weight, the chances are you are not going to stick to it.

I was previously a swimmer and, as a teenager, I never viewed my swim training as exercise or a way to achieve a certain physique. I viewed it as a social club where I made friends, as a competitive sport, as a hobby – and it was fun. Don't get me wrong, the training was hard going, but I enjoyed it. This is why I also enjoy weight training in the gym because it is a challenge for me mentally and physically – and I can push myself to do things I couldn't do before. Of course, I do train a certain way to gain aesthetic benefits from my work at the gym but that is not my only reason for going.

Exercise is often sold to us as a way to lose weight, burn calories and get in shape for summer. But, to really benefit long-term from exercising, it is important to shift your mindset and focus on all of the other health benefits it can provide. Focusing too much on weight loss and aesthetic goals can have negative effects on how you perceive exercise and will impact on the duration for which you actually stick with it. Thinking of exercise simply as a means of weight loss can lead us to feel guilty if we do not stick to our exercise regime – and this guilt can result in over exercising and restricted eating behaviours. In addition, it is typically found that the majority of individuals who do lose weight via exercise will regain it again because they are more likely to stop exercising when they attain their 'target weight'.

Yo-yo dieting can have detrimental effects on both our mental health and physical health; thus focusing purely on weight loss as a reason for exercise can actually have negative effects on our overall health. Physicians often tell patients to work out to lose weight, lower cholesterol or prevent illness such as diabetes. Unfortunately, it can take months before any physical results of your hard work in the gym are apparent, which means that many people give up on exercise.

With this in mind, let's shift the conversation around exercise onto to the many other benefits it can provide. You don't have to be a fitness fanatic to reap the rewards of working out. Research has suggested that small amounts of exercise can make a significant difference across all ages and fitness levels.

1. MOOD

It is no secret that you never regret a workout. Exercise increases endorphin levels, which are natural mood lifters meaning you will feel good after your workout. As well as releasing endorphins in the brain, physical activity helps to relax the muscles and relieve tension in the body. Since the body and mind are so closely linked, when your body feels better so, too, will your mind. Within five minutes of moderate exercise, your mood will become more positive; but the effects of physical activity on mental wellbeing extend beyond the short-term. Research shows that exercise can also help alleviate long-term depression.

2. SHARPER MEMORY AND THINKING

The same endorphins that improve your mood also help you concentrate. Some researchers believe exercise alleviates depression by increasing serotonin (the neurotransmitter targeted by antidepressants), or brain-derived neurotrophic factor (which supports the growth of neurons). Another theory suggests exercise helps by normalising sleep, which is known to have protective effects on the brain.

3. IMPROVED SLEEP

Sleep. My favourite word! I personally feel the effects of the exercise and sleep relationship. If I take more than two days off from exercise, I start to feel restless at night and find it much harder to fall asleep. Even small amounts of exercise in the morning or afternoon can help to regulate your sleeping patterns.

4. IMPROVED SELF-ESTEEM

Regular exercise is an investment in your mind, body and soul. By meeting small exercise goals, you will feel a sense of achievement. Taking time for yourself is extremely important and dedicating even ten minutes a day to go for a walk, do some stretching or yoga can have huge benefits. If you begin thinking of physical activity as a priority, you will soon find ways to fit small amounts into a busy schedule.

5. MORE ENERGY

When you're tired or stressed out from daily life, it sometimes feels like working out will just make it worse. You know the feeling of finishing work and having the dreaded gym session lying ahead? But the truth is that exercise is a powerful energiser. Studies show that regular exercise can reduce fatigue and increase your energy levels.

GETTING STARTED

Usually the hardest part of exercising is actually getting started. It is important to first establish where you are in your fitness journey and make realistic goals for yourself. I see so many new gym members in January and by February they are nowhere to be seen. They start off too hard and get burnt out and end up with a negative relationship with exercise. If you are new to exercise, let's be realistic: it's unlikely that going to the gym five times a week and smashing the weights will be for you. Having said that, if it is something you want to get into, you most certainly can: you just have to start off slowly and build it up over time.

My five top tips to getting started and staying motivated are ...

1. FOCUS ON ACTIVITIES YOU ENJOY

The gym isn't for everyone, but exercise is! Whether you enjoy going on walks or hikes with friends, swimming, dancing, cycling, yoga, weightlifting, cross fit; do what works for you. I grew up swimming and I loved it, now my new love is weight training in the gym. This book shares some of my favourite at home and gym workouts for you to try if you want to get into that area of fitness. However, it is really important that you do what you love. If you do something you genuinely enjoy, you are more likely to stick to it!

2. MAKE EXERCISE PART OF YOUR LIFESTYLE

In a similar way, to eating healthily, make exercise a part of your lifestyle. If you look at healthy eating and exercise as a chore and a diet, then you are not going to stick to it. Cultivate a positive attitude towards eating healthy food and working out and think of all of the non-physical benefits having a healthy lifestyle can offer – think how good you will feel after finishing off a workout and drinking a delicious homemade smoothie! It is important to make working out fit into your lifestyle so if the morning works for you, then go to the gym in the morning. If you love yoga and the only time you can go is 8 p.m. on a Monday, then book that class!

3. REWARD YOURSELF

Part of the reward of completing an activity is how much better you'll feel afterwards, but it always helps your motivation to do something for yourself. Whether this is a daily bubble bath post-workout or if you hit your exercise goals for the week and have an at home spa day with all your favourite products while catching up on your favourite TV shows. Making weekly workout goals and noting them in your fitness journal to tick off at the end of the week is a great way to see what you have accomplished. It is important to start small. It is important to take manageable steps. Mark small successes along the way so you feel good and don't get discouraged by setting expectations too high too soon. Start by writing down a daily or weekly goal and decide when you will increase it.

4. MAKE EXERCISE A SOCIAL ACTIVITY

Grab a friend to work out with – it'll make exercise more fun and enjoyable, but also help motivate you to stick to a workout routine. Look up your favourite workout to do together or book your favourite class to attend at the gym. Accountability is so helpful – you wouldn't cancel on your friend, now, would you?

5. PLAN AHEAD

Everyone is busy and this is the easiest excuse on the planet to get out of doing your workout. Plan your week ahead so you know what days you want to work out and plan each workout, so you know what you are doing each day. Taking just thirty minutes to do this on a Sunday night will help you to see your week more clearly and stick to your goals. The back of this book has a weekly workout schedule which I created so you can see exactly how you might like to arrange your week.

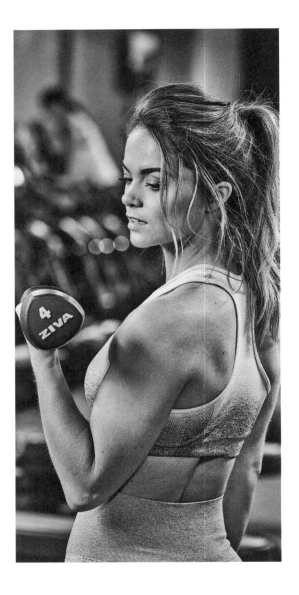

A WORD ON WEIGHTS

My fitness journey has led me to weight training and I absolutely love it. There is, however, still a stigma around women and weight training as people mistakenly believe that lifting weights will automatically make you bulky – which is an aesthetic not everyone wants to achieve. I can understand why weight training might seem off-putting: the slamming of weights, weird noises and grunts, overall not having a clue what to do – it's overwhelming.

Typically, yes, the weights room seems to be full of men . . . but I think this might be to do with the old stereotype that muscles are reserved only for men. This isn't the case! Weight training can be one of the most beneficial forms of exercise for anyone of any age in terms of looking and feeling great. Muscles are for everyone.

For me personally, weight training has helped me shape my body and love myself more. For those women concerned that their bodies might look less 'feminine' if they weight train, my experience has been that I've only enhanced my not-so-naturally-there curves.

I think what people fail to realise when it comes to exercise is that weight loss and fat loss are two different things. For me, I have never needed to lose weight, but I have wanted to build more of a shape and lose fat. That is, to build lean muscle mass and lose fat to have an overall athletic shape. Weight training allowed me to do that. Strength and resistance training builds muscle, which has a higher metabolic rate than fat. This means that your resting metabolic rate – your energy expenditure – is higher if you have more muscle than body fat.

Strength training has also led to me feeling more confident in everyday life; not just in terms of how I look but how I feel. Being physically strong is empowering . . . my favourite activity is getting on an aeroplane and being the one to help others lift their bags into the overhead lockers!

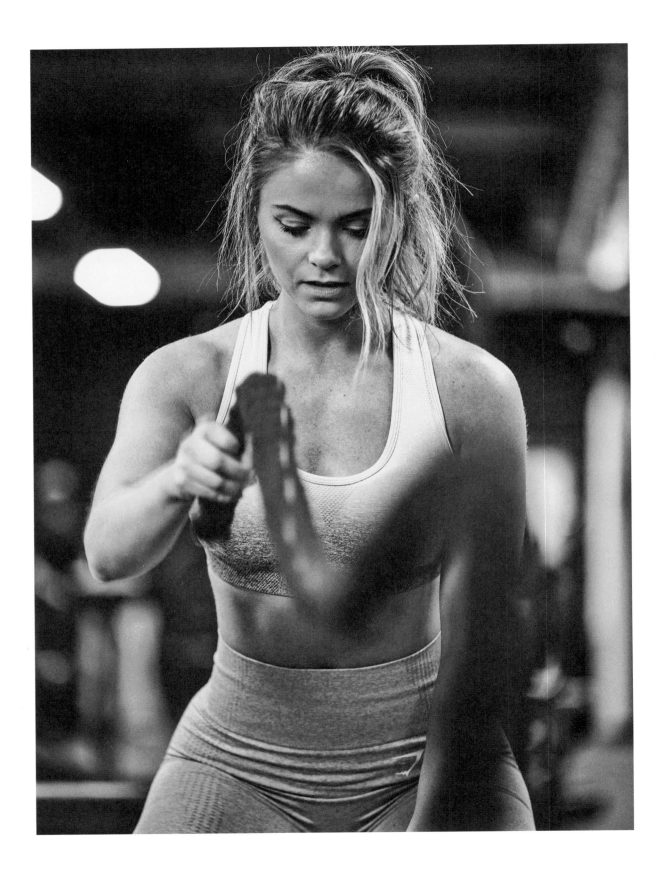

GYM-BASED WORKOUT PLAN

The focus of this fitness plan is weight training – let's talk about why. Weights are amazing for sculpting the body. They allow you to grow lean muscle while simultaneously burning fat. However, weight training only works when it's done properly. Every day, I see people in the gym just going through the motions with little to no effort, no clue what they are doing or why, not engaging the right muscles. We do not want this to be you.

Weight training is amazing if you do it properly. If you are completely new to weights, then please:

- Use this book.
- Watch exercise videos online.
- Go to your gym and ask a trainer or gym instructor if your form is correct.

Remember – effort is required! The rep ranges for these workouts are in the hypertrophy-specific range – which is what causes muscle growth. This range is anything from 8 to 20 reps. Optimal range is 8 to 15. Here, I recommend between 10 to 15 reps for most exercises, performing between 3 to 5 sets per exercise.

In this plan you will find four gym-based workouts to complete across the week; two upper body and two lower body workouts. The first upper body workout combines chest, triceps and shoulders for a 'push' workout. The second upper body workout combines back and biceps for a 'pull' workout. Combining muscle groups in this way means you can train them more frequently – for example, my weekly workout schedule is push, pull, legs, push, pull, legs, meaning I train all body parts twice in one week.

Now, this does mean I weight train six times per week – this is advanced and not recommended for beginners. Beginners should either start with the four workouts outlined below or even drop one of the leg days to start with three days per week and then build from there. It is important to spread your training out across the week, so beginners could aim to go to the gym Monday, Wednesday and Fridays to start with.

This also allows you to use the other four days for activities you already enjoy such as that yoga or dance class you love on a Saturday morning! These other days also allow you to rest and recover (grow your new baby muscles). The idea of this book is to help enhance your life and your body; to help you look and feel your happiest and strongest – overdoing any part of your new routine will end up having the opposite effect.

OPTIMISING YOUR WORKOUT

1. START WHERE YOU ARE

There is no point jumping in the deep end if you can't swim. If you are a complete beginner take these workouts and add them to your weekly schedule when it suits YOUR lifestyle. Start with three workouts per week to get into the routine and get familiar with this new style of exercise. You will be able to build on this and advance over time; remember slow and steady wins the race. That leads me neatly to my second tip.

2. PROGRESS IS SLOW

Don't be that guy that eats one healthy meal and does one workout and expects to wake up the next day looking like a *Baywatch* lifeguard. That is unrealistic. You know the saying, 'Rome wasn't built in a day'? Well, it took you your whole life to get to where you are now, so it is going to take you more than a week to get to where you want to be. So . . .

3. ENJOY YOUR JOURNEY!

The point of *Naturally Stefanie* is to create a healthy, sustainable lifestyle; this is not a fad diet or weight loss book. I'm in danger of repeating myself, but I LOVE training and I love it because it is a never-ending journey: there is no final destination that you will reach and finally be 'happy'. You have to enjoy each workout and each healthy meal and know you are doing good for your body, not punishing it. Don't work out to counteract what you have eaten; use what you have eaten to fuel your workout. That is the mindset I would love you to have. Learn to push your body to see what it can achieve; every small achievement is an achievement.

4. FOCUS ON THE PROCESS

I remember the first time I could bench press the bar . . . without additional weight, just the bar. For me, 20 kilos was very heavy and I had to start off with the lightest of dumbbells before I could progress onto the 'big boys' bench. Now I can do more than three times that weight, and bench press more than my own bodyweight. Crazy right? But it took me over four years. Enjoy the process – don't worry too much about the outcome.

WARMING UP

Over the next few pages you will see the warm-up exercises that I advise you to perform before each workout. These warm-up exercises are really important. They will ensure you reduce your chances of injury and will improve your recovery time.

Now that you are all motivated to start your new workout routine here are a few things to keep in mind.

1. BODY WEIGHT IS GREAT

If you are a beginner, start with the body weight exercise variations of the exercises outlined in the workouts. From there, start with the lightest weights in the dumbbell section and on the machines to gauge your strength and your starting point.

Now, some of you might just be naturally strong and be able to lift a reasonable amount, but the reality is most of you will have to start with the lightest weights or even just your body weight. THIS IS FINE!

2. WORK THOSE WEIGHTS

To find your 'working weight' (the weight you are going to use effectively for the exercise one that is neither too heavy nor too light), find the weight that you can perform between 8 to 12 repetitions with while maintaining proper form.

3. REST MATTERS

Listen to your body and take rest between exercises. Go by how you feel, but I usually recommend rests of between one to two minutes between sets and exercises. For example, perform your first set of squats,

rest for one to two minutes, perform the second and so on. Once you have completed all of the necessary sets for this exercise, move onto the next.

4. VARIATIONS ON A THEME

If your gym does not have some of the equipment that the workouts suggest, simply ask an instructor for a variation or look up one online; the aim is to work the target muscle, and this can be done in multiple ways! Similarly, if you find using barbells too heavy you can do dumbbell variations of the exercises to get you started and build up your strength first.

5. IF IN DOUBT, ASK!

If you are unsure of how to do any of the exercises or want to have your form checked out, ask an instructor in the gym; it's what they are there for! The last thing you want to do is injure yourself on day one and have a fear of going back to the gym again.

If you would like more help and advice on the workouts in this book, my vegan fitness site, Vegan Aesthetics, provides seasonal 12-week workout guides to thousands of members worldwide. It offers support for both gym and home-based workouts, and will help keep you on track!

WORKOUTS

DAY 1

PUSH – SHOULDERS, CHEST & TRICEPS
WARM-UP EXERCISES

SETS	REPS		
3	10–15	Arm circles	
3	10–15	Across body arm swings	
3	10–15	Press-ups on knees	
3	10–15	Very light dumbbell chest press	
3	10–15	Very light seated dumbbell shoulder press	

BENCH PRESS TECHNIQUE

Be sure to get your bench press technique spot on.
Avoid 'flat back' benching – it's a really common error that
will damage your shoulders.

PUSH – SHOULDERS, CHEST & TRICEPS
WORKOUT EXERCISES

EXERCISE	SETS	REPS	
1	3	8–12	Bench press
2	3	12–15	Standing dumbbell press
3	3	12–15	Machine chest press
4	3	12–15 per arm	Seated lateral raises
5	3	15–20 per arm	Dumbbell rear delt flies
6	3	15–20 per side	Oblique cable twists
7	3	10–12	Tricep dips

EXERCISE 1 – BENCH PRESS

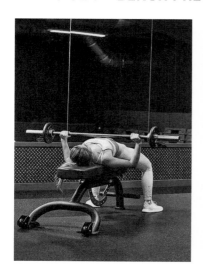 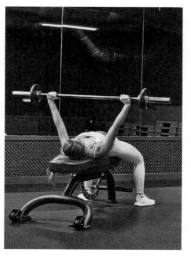 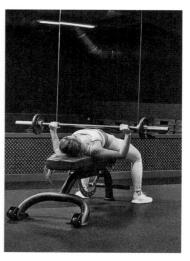

EXERCISE 2 – STANDING DUMBBELL PRESS

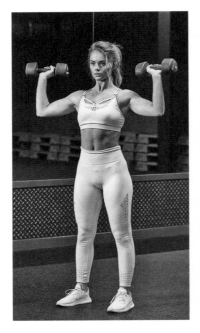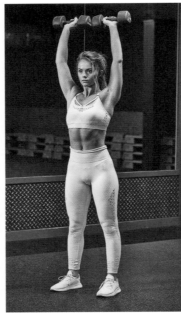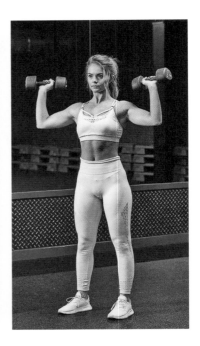

EXERCISE 3 – MACHINE CHEST PRESS

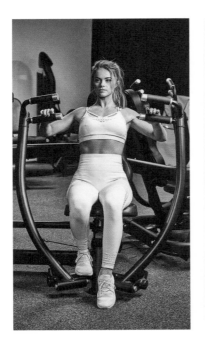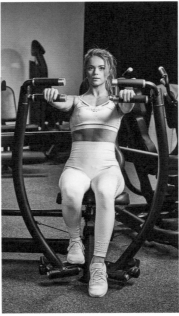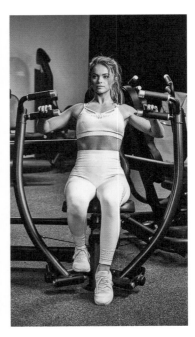

EXERCICE 4
SEATED LATERAL RAISES

EXERCISE 5
DUMBBELL REAR DELT FLIES

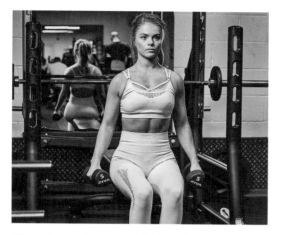

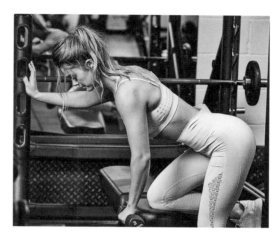

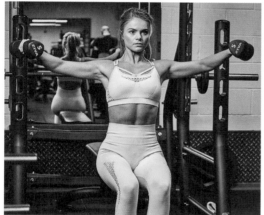

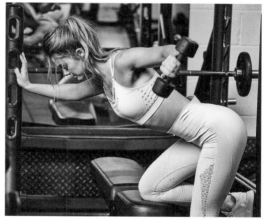

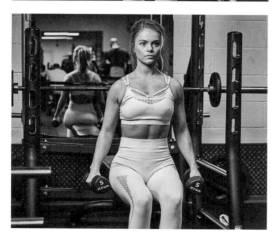

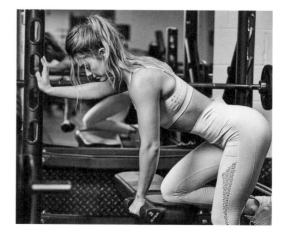

WORKOUTS

EXERCISE 6
OBLIQUE CABLE TWISTS

EXERCISE 7
TRICEP DIPS

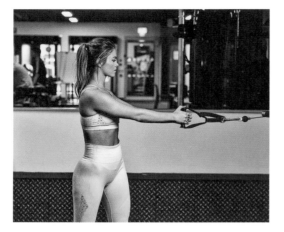

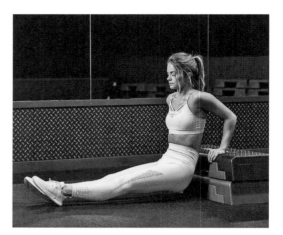

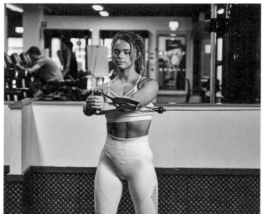

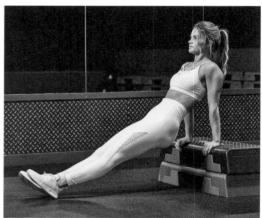

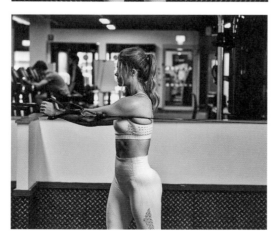

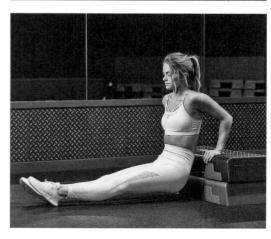

. . . are a great body weight exercise to sculpt the back
of your arms. Don't be fooled, they are a lot harder than they look.
Practise them and you will soon feel invincible!

DAY 2

LEG – QUADS, GLUTES & HAMSTRINGS
WARM-UP EXERCISES

SETS	REPS	
3	10–15	Bodyweight squats
3	10–15	Bodyweight walking lunges
3	10–15	Bodyweight donkey kicks
3	10–15	Very light barbell or dumbbell squats

LEG – QUADS, GLUTES & HAMSTRINGS
WORKOUT EXERCISES

EXERCISE	SETS	REPS	
1	3	8–12	Squats
2	3	10–15	Hip thrusts
3	3	10–12 per leg	Split leg lunges
4	3	15–20 per leg	Cable kickbacks
5	3	12–15	Machine hamstring curls
6	3	30 sec to 1 minute	Plank

EXERCISE 1 – SQUATS

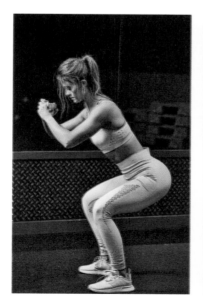 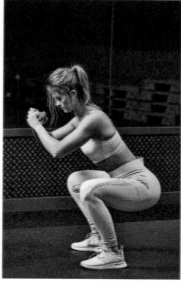 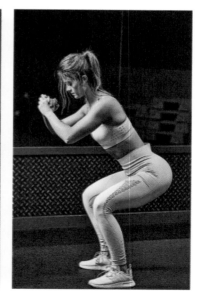

EXERCISE 2
HIP THRUSTS

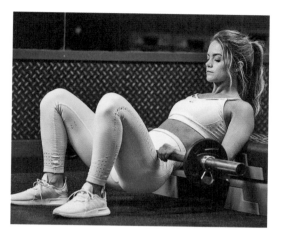

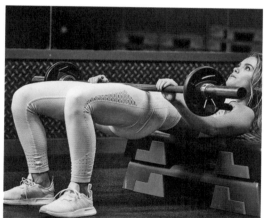

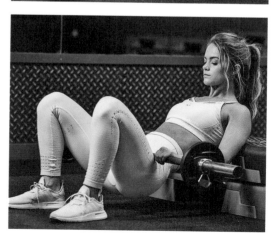

EXERCISE 3
SPLIT LEG LUNGES

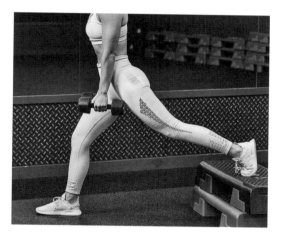

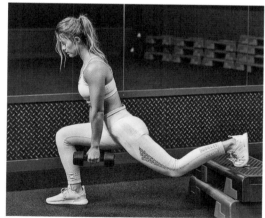

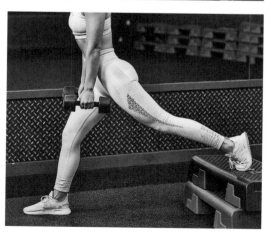

WORKOUTS

EXERCISE 4
CABLE KICKBACKS

EXERCISE 5
MACHINE HAMSTRING CURLS

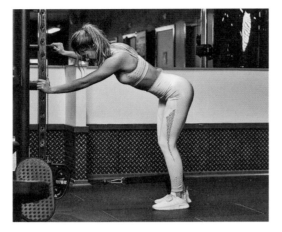

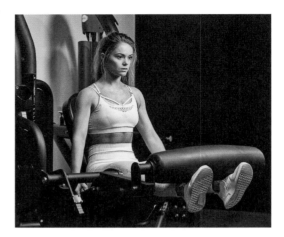

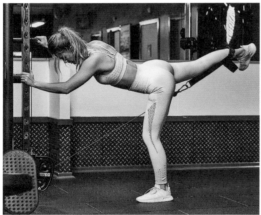

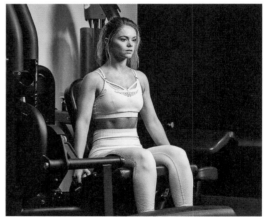

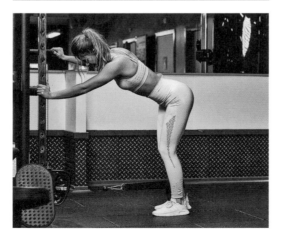

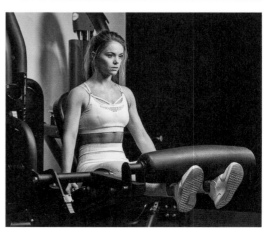

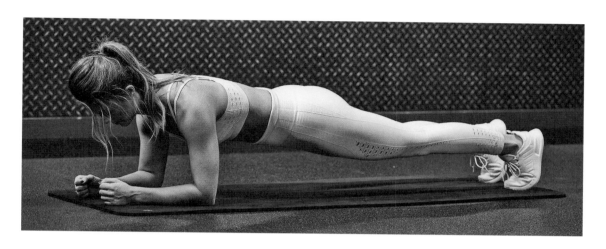

DAY 3

PULL – BACK & BICEPS
WARM-UP EXERCISES

SETS	REPS	
3	10–15	Arm circles
3	10–15	Across body arm swings
3	10–15	Assisted pull-ups
3	10–15	Very light barbell rows

PULL – BACK & BICEPS
WORKOUT EXERCISES

EXERCISE	SETS	REPS	
1	3	10–15	Barbell bend over rows
2	3	12–15 per arm	Single arm seated cable rows
3	3	12–15	EZ bar curls
4	3	10–12	Wide grip lat pull-downs
5	3	12–15	Cable rope curls
6	3	3–5, hold for 30 sec	Hanging leg raises

EXERCISE 1 – BARBELL BEND OVER ROWS

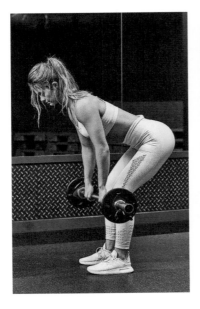
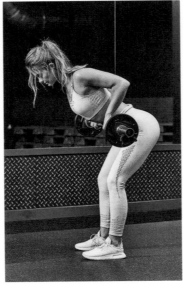
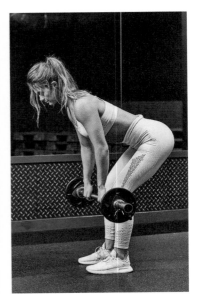

EXERCISE 2 – SINGLE ARM SEATED CABLE ROWS

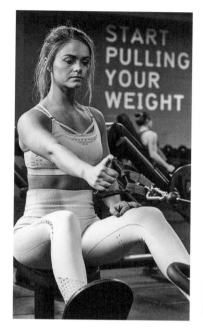 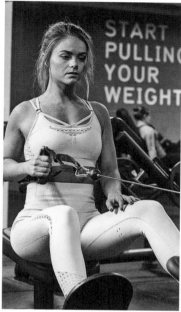 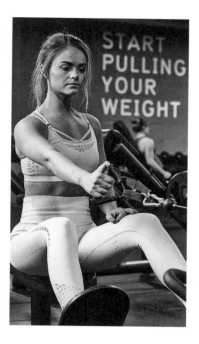

EXERCISE 3 – EZ BAR CURLS

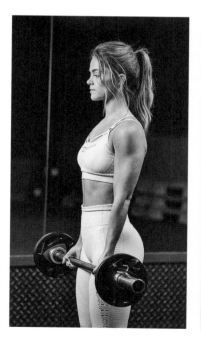 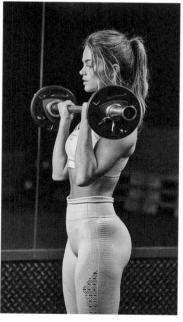 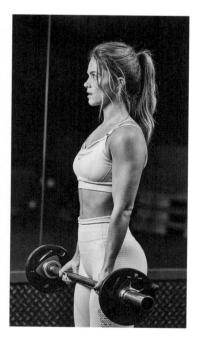

EXERCISE 4 – **WIDE GRIP LAT PULL-DOWNS**

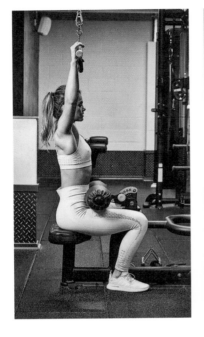 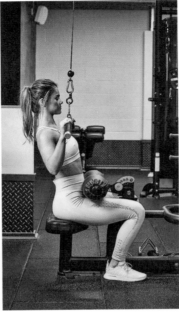 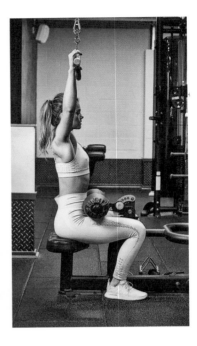

EXERCISE 5 – **CABLE ROPE CURLS**

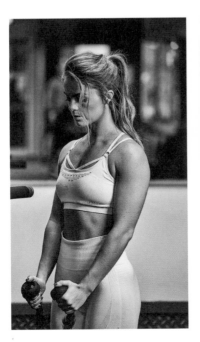 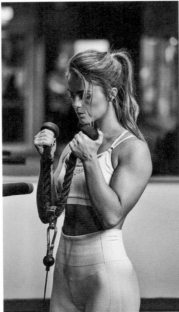 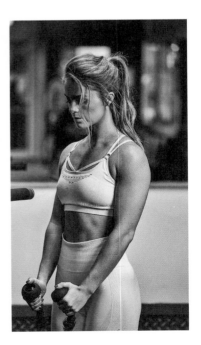

EXERCISE 6 – HANGING LEG RAISES

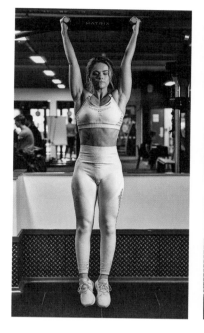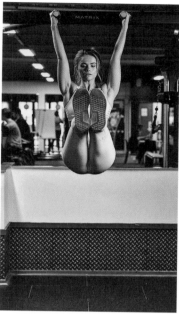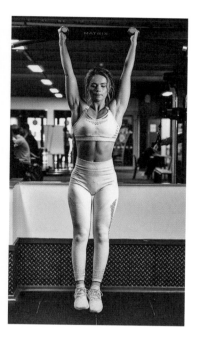

BUILD A CORE . . .

. . . of steel with hanging leg raises. But always perform this seriously impressive exercise with total control. The idea is NOT to swing your legs to lift them!

DAY 4

LEG – QUADS, GLUTES & HAMSTRINGS
WARM-UP EXERCISES

SETS	REPS		
3	10–15	Bodyweight squats	
3	10–15	Bodyweight walking lunges	
3	10–15	Bodyweight donkey kicks	
3	10–15	Very light barbell or dumbbell squats	

LEG – QUADS, GLUTES & HAMSTRINGS
WORKOUT EXERCISES

EXERCISE	SETS	REPS		
1	3	8–12	Deadlifts	
2	3	10–12 per leg	Walking lunges	
3	3	10–12	Goblet squats	
4	3	12–15	Dumbbell RDL	
5	3	15–20	Machine leg extensions	
6	3	10–15 per side	Bicycle crunches	

EXERCISE 1 – DEADLIFTS

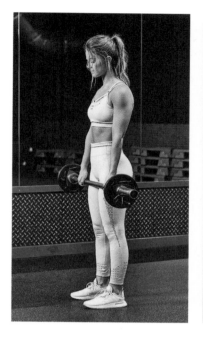
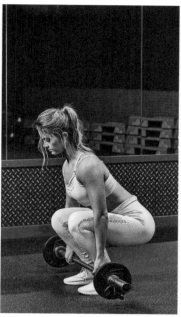
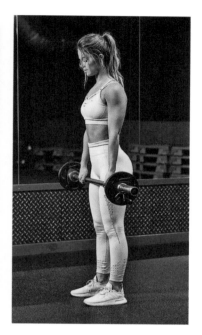

EXERCISE 2 – WALKING LUNGES

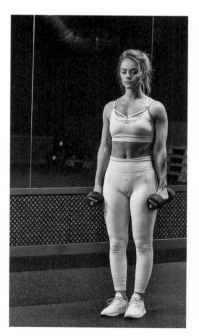
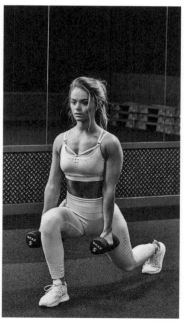
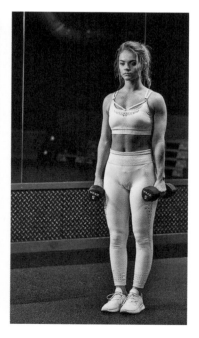

EXERCISE 3 – GOBLET SQUATS

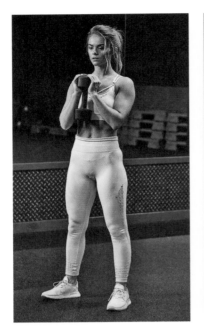 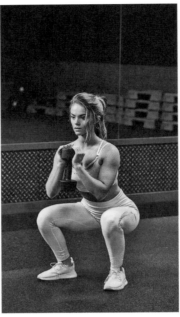 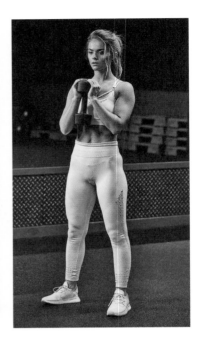

EXERCISE 4 – DUMBBELL RDL (ROMANIAN DEADLIFTS)

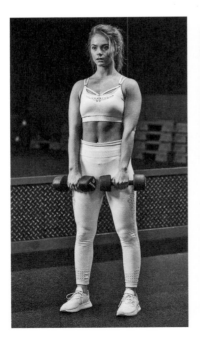 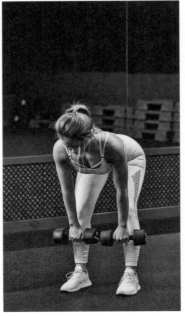 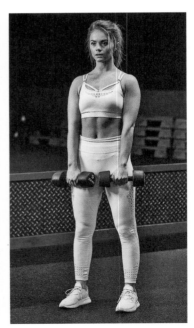

EXERCISE 5
MACHINE LEG EXTENSIONS

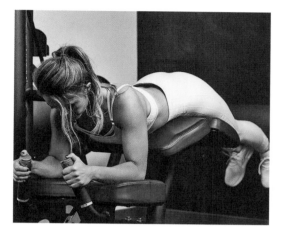

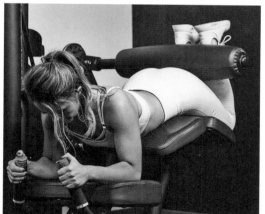

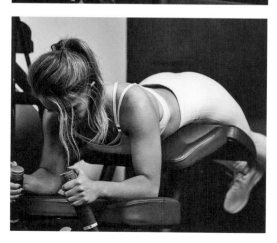

EXERCISE 6
BICYCLE CRUNCHES

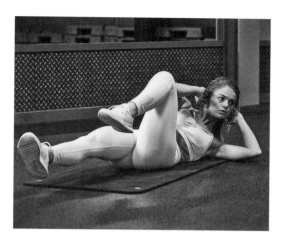

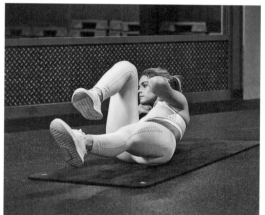

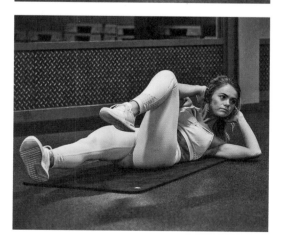

HOME WORKOUT PLAN

YOU WILL NEED

1. Adjustable dumbbells
2. Exercise mat

The home workout plan is an at home variation of the gym plan and allows you to work out from the comfort of your own home. The style of the workouts is a little different. There are four workouts in this plan; two upper body and two lower body which replicate the exercises from the gym plan but use only bodyweight and dumbbells.

WORKOUTS

There are 10 exercises per workout which are split into 2 circuits of 5 exercises. Perform each exercise in the first circuit for 30 seconds and do each of the 5 exercises back to back until you have completed a 2.5 minute circuit.

Rest for 1 minute and repeat the first circuit 3 times. Repeat this with the second circuit. This will give you a total workout time of 15 minutes with 6 minutes of rest in between. Your workout will be complete in around 20 minutes.

SQUAT JUMPS WILL TAKE . . .

. . . your training to the next level. Push yourself and this great cardio exercise will build explosive power.

DAY 1

LEGS
CIRCUIT 1

EXERCISE	TIME	
1	30 seconds	Squat jumps
2	30 seconds	Side lunges
3	30 seconds	Single leg glute bridge left
4	30 seconds	Single leg glute bridge right
5	30 seconds	Goblet squats

EXERCISE 1 – **SQUAT JUMPS**

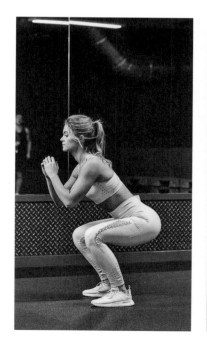
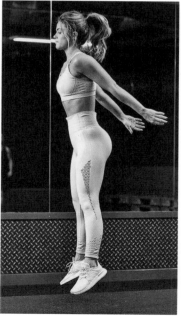
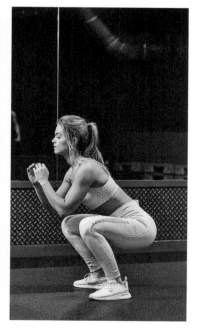

WORKOUTS

EXERCISE 2 – **SIDE LUNGES**

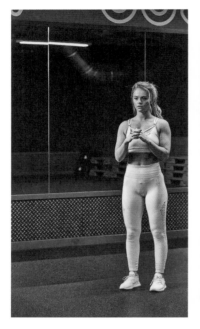 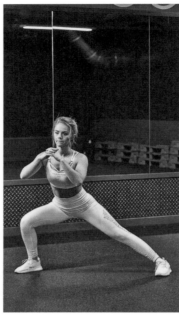 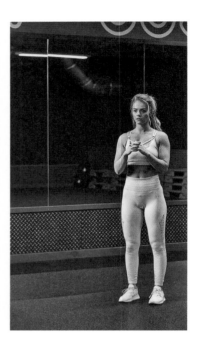

EXERCISE 3 – **SINGLE LEG GLUTE BRIDGE LEFT**

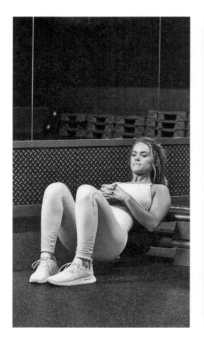 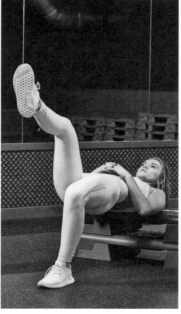 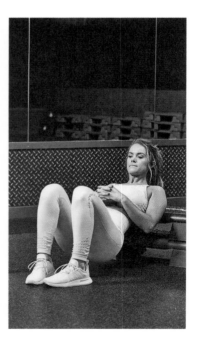

EXERCISE 4 – **SINGLE LEG GLUTE BRIDGE RIGHT**

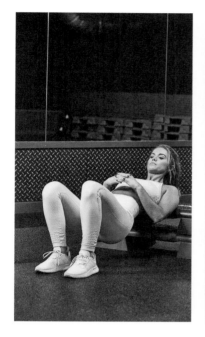 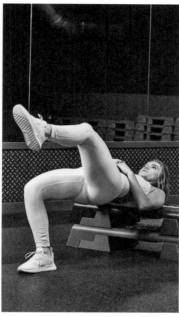 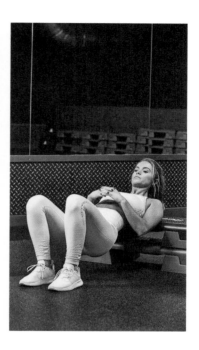

EXERCISE 5 – **GOBLET SQUATS**

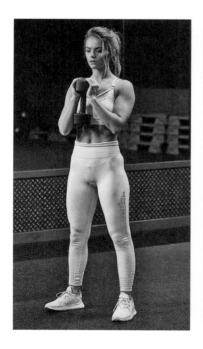 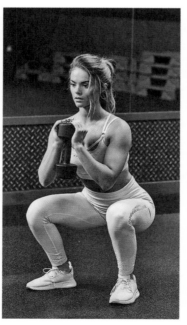 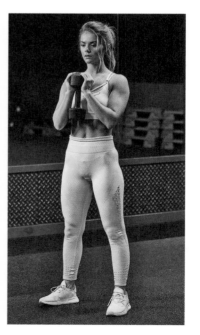

LEGS
CIRCUIT 2

EXERCISE	TIME	
1	30 seconds	Dumbbell stiff leg deadlifts
2	30 seconds	Sumo squats with dumbbell
3	30 seconds	Double glute bridge
4	30 seconds	Pulse lunges left leg
5	30 seconds	Pulse lunges right leg

EXERCISE 1 – DUMBBELL STIFF LEG DEADLIFTS

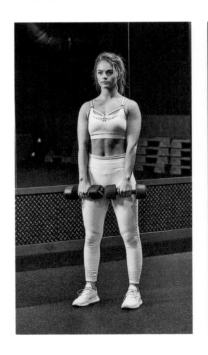 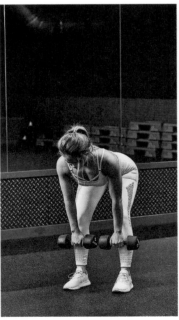 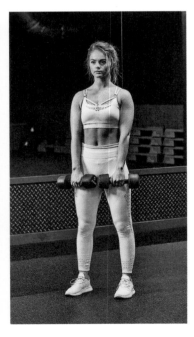

EXERCISE 2
SUMO SQUATS WITH DUMBBELL

EXERCISE 3
DOUBLE GLUTE BRIDGE

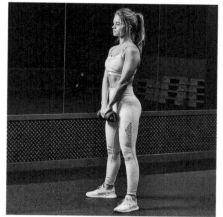

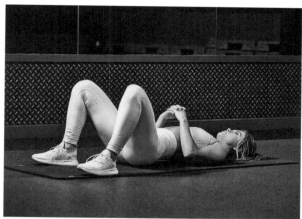

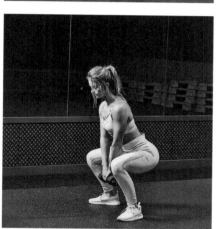

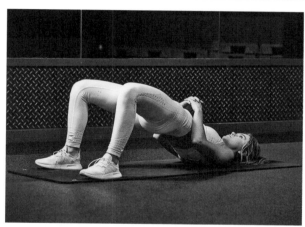

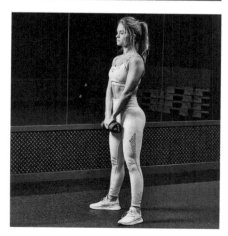

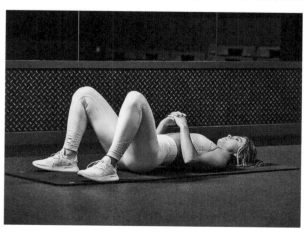

EXERCISE 4 – PULSE LUNGES LEFT LEG

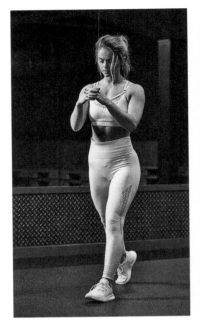 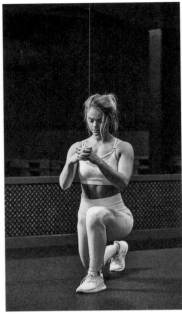 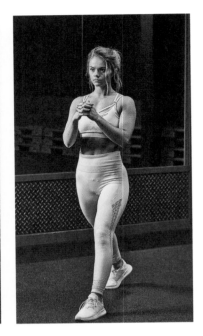

EXERCISE 5 – PULSE LUNGES RIGHT LEG

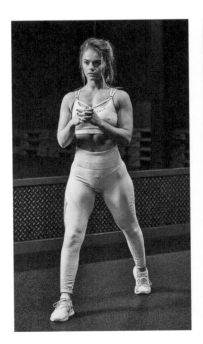 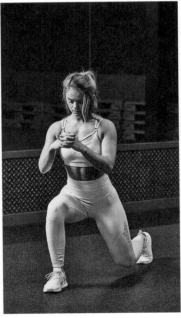 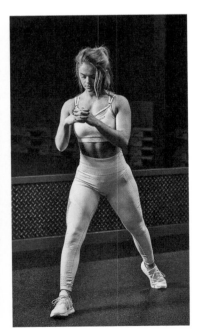

DAY 2

UPPER BODY
CIRCUIT 1

EXERCISE	TIME	
1	30 seconds	Mountain climbers
2	30 seconds	Dumbbell rows left arm
3	30 seconds	Dumbbell rows right arm
4	30 seconds	Bicycle crunches
5	30 seconds	Supermans

WORKOUTS

EXERCISE 1
MOUNTAIN CLIMBERS

EXERCISE 2
DUMBBELL ROWS LEFT ARM

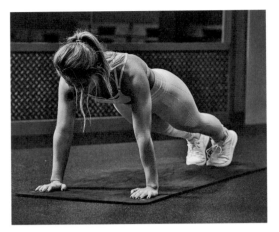

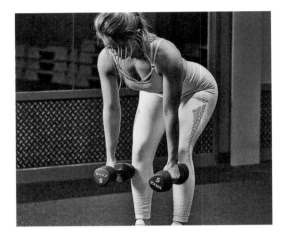

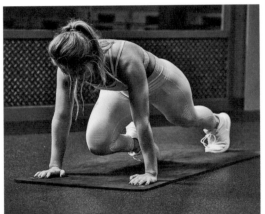

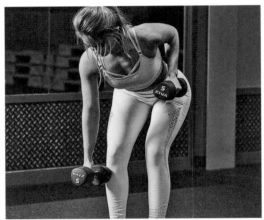

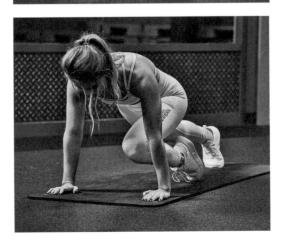

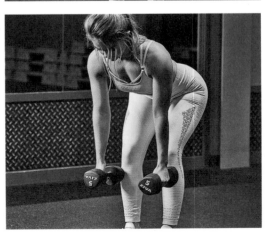

EXERCISE 3
DUMBBELL ROWS RIGHT ARM

EXERCISE 4
BICYCLE CRUNCHES

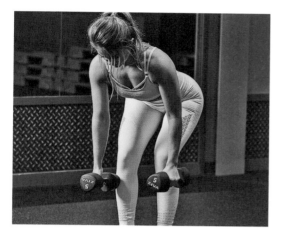

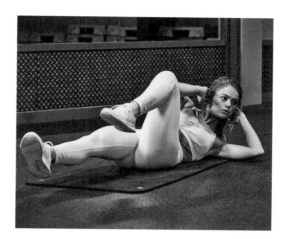

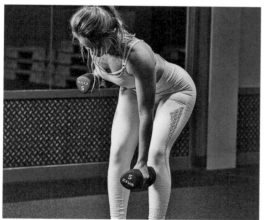

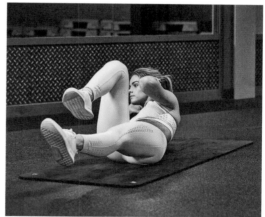

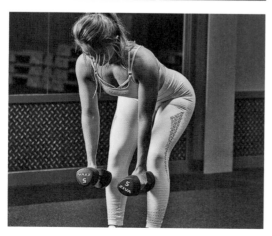

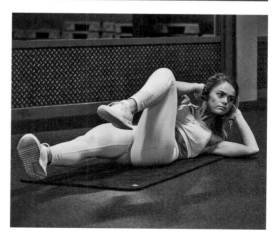

EXERCISE 5
SUPERMANS

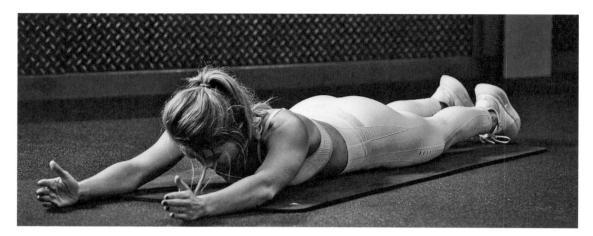

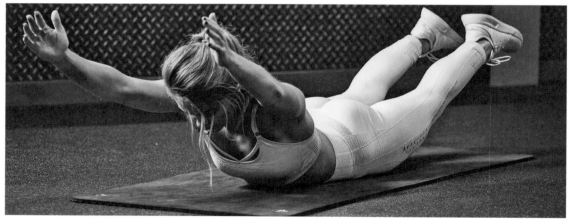

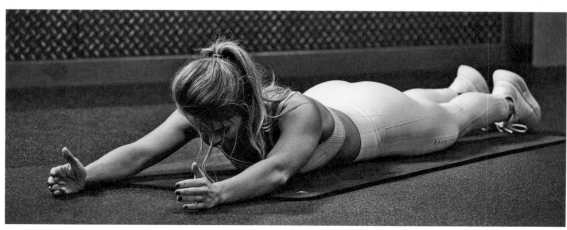

UPPER BODY
CIRCUIT 2

EXERCISE	TIME	
1	30 seconds	Plank rows
2	30 seconds	Standing dumbbell press
3	30 seconds	Dumbbell supinate curls
4	30 seconds	Scissor kicks
5	30 seconds	Plank in and outs

EXERCISE 1 – PLANK ROWS

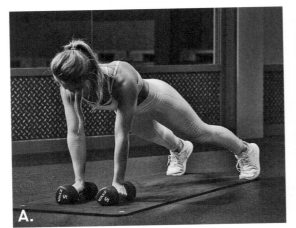

A.

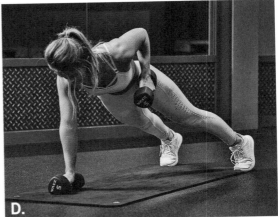

D.

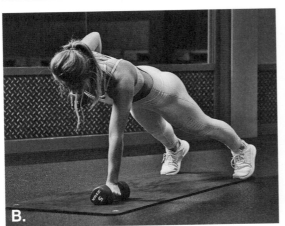

B.

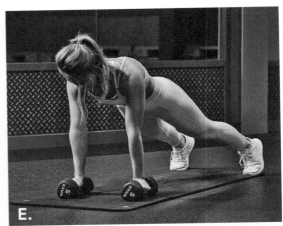

E.

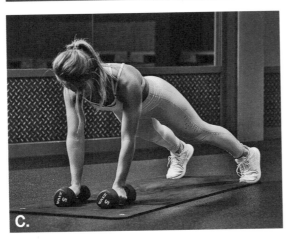

C.

EXERCISE 2 – STANDING DUMBBELL PRESS

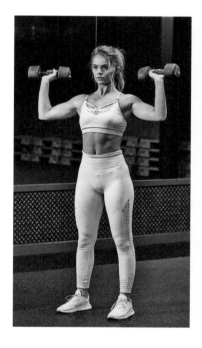 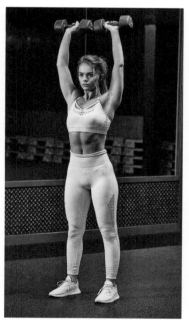 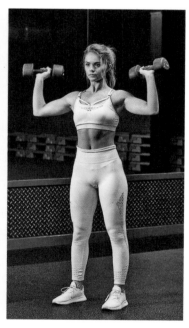

EXERCISE 3 – DUMBBELL SUPINATE CURLS

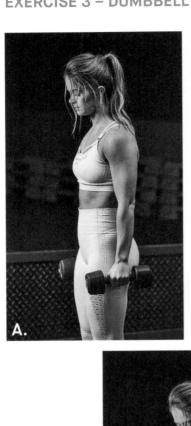

A.

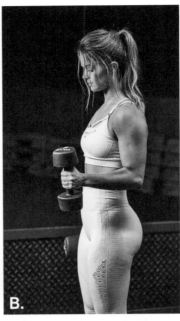

B.

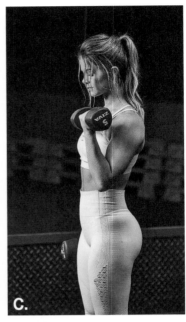

C.

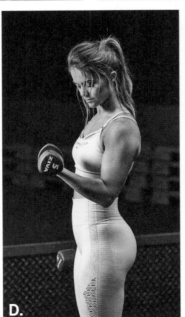

D.

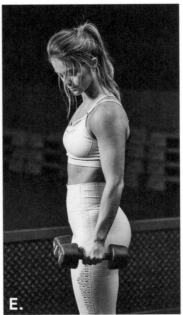

E.

EXERCISE 4– SCISSOR KICKS

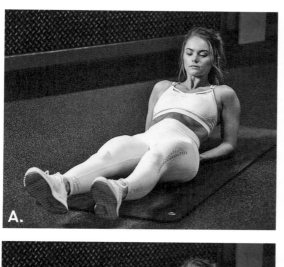

A.

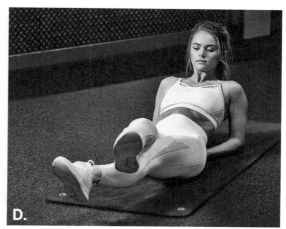

D.

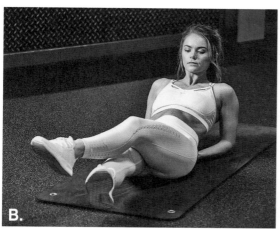

B.

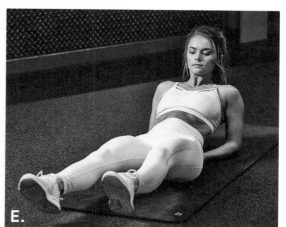

E.

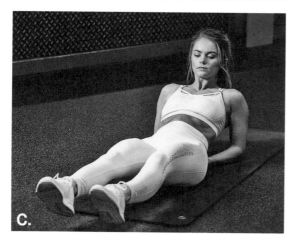

C.

EXERCISE 5 – PLANK IN AND OUTS

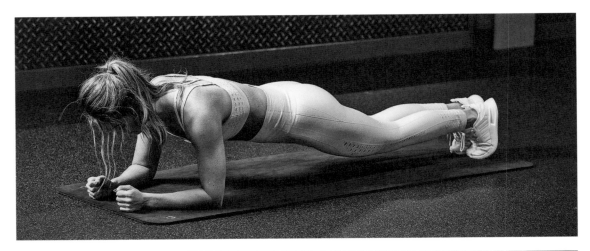

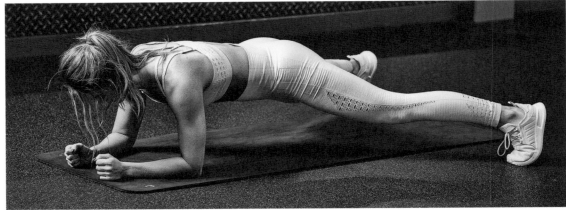

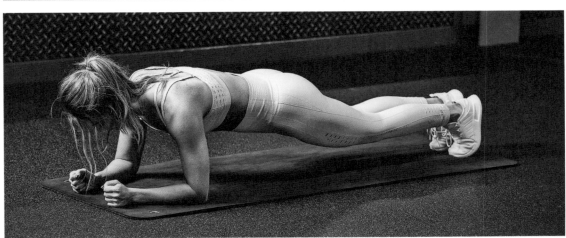

DAY 3

LEGS
CIRCUIT 1

EXERCISE	TIME	
1	30 seconds	Cross body jump squats
2	30 seconds	Dumbbell pulse squats (stay low)
3	30 seconds	Scissor jump squats
4	30 seconds	Alternating drop lunges
5	30 seconds	Wall sit

EXERCISE 1 – CROSS BODY JUMP SQUATS

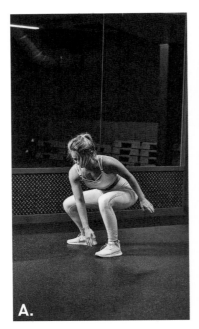

A.

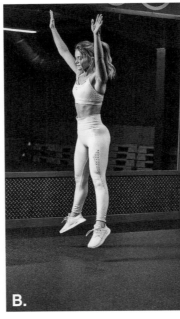

B.

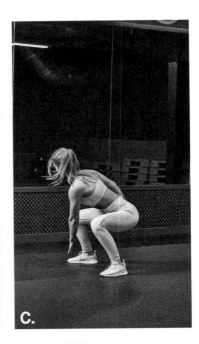

C.

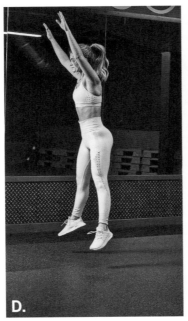

D.

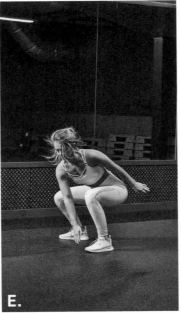

E.

EXERCISE 2 – DUMBBELL PULSE SQUATS (STAY LOW)

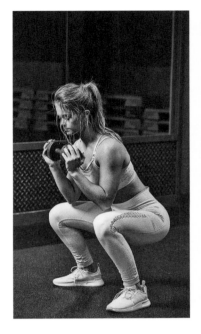 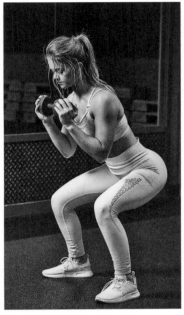 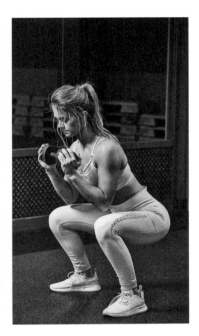

EXERCISE 3 – SCISSOR JUMP SQUATS

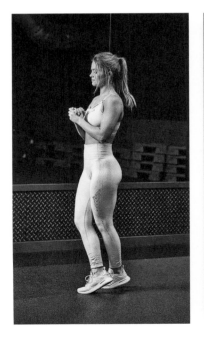 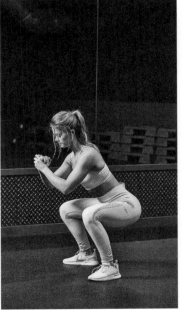 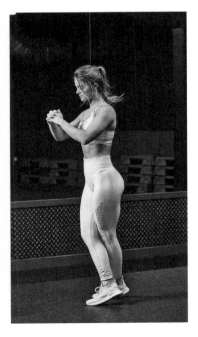

EXERCISE 4 – **ALTERNATING DROP LUNGES**   EXERCISE 5 – **WALL SIT**

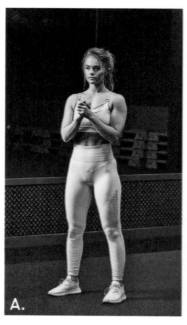

A.

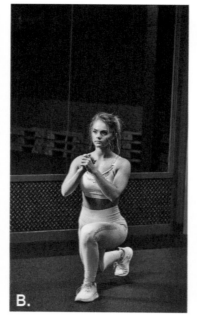

B.

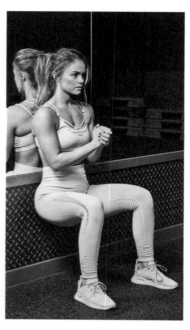

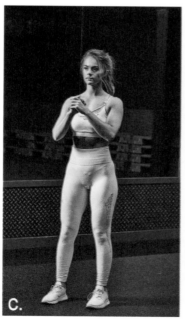

C.

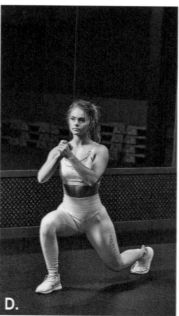

D.

LEGS
CIRCUIT 2

EXERCISE	TIME	
1	30 seconds	Pulse squats
2	30 seconds	Squat walk
3	30 seconds	Lunges with knee lift
4	30 seconds	Dumbbell calf raises left
5	30 seconds	Dumbbell calf raises right

EXERCISE 1 – PULSE SQUATS

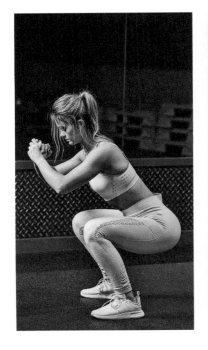
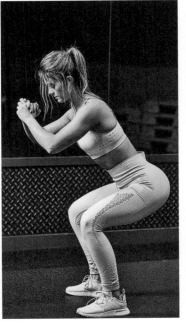
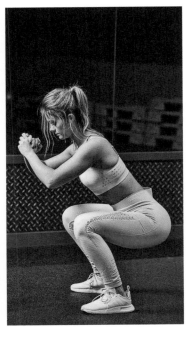

EXERCISE 2 – SQUAT WALK

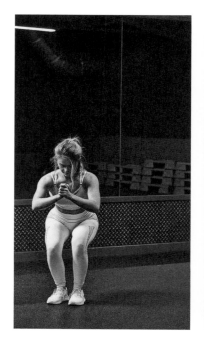
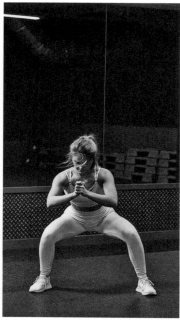
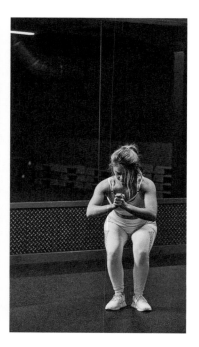

EXERCISE 3 – LUNGES WITH KNEE LIFT

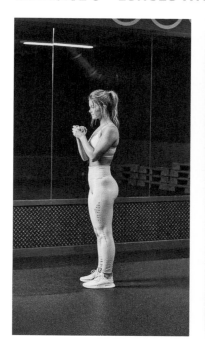
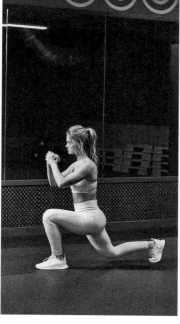
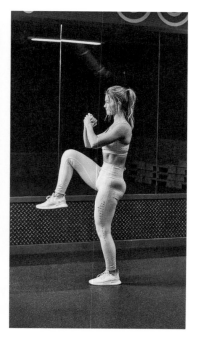

EXERCISE 4 – DUMBBELL CALF RAISES LEFT

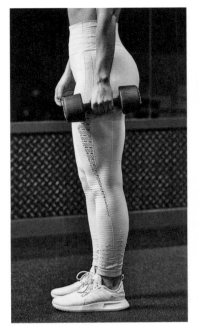 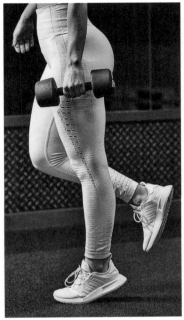 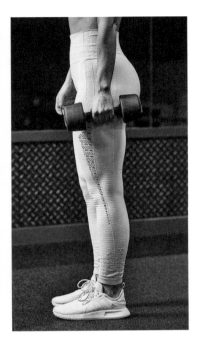

EXERCISE 5 – DUMBBELL CALF RAISES RIGHT

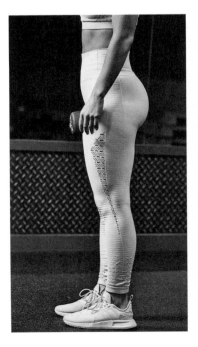 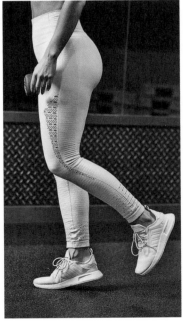 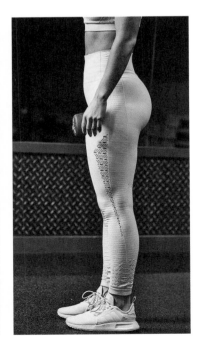

DAY 4

SHOULDERS, CHEST & TRICEPS
CIRCUIT 1

EXERCICE	TIME		
1	30 seconds	Press-ups	
2	30 seconds	Dumbbell chest press	
3	30 seconds	Dumbbell flies	
4	30 seconds	Seated shoulder press	
5	30 seconds	Wide grip push-ups	

EXERCISE 1 – PRESS-UPS

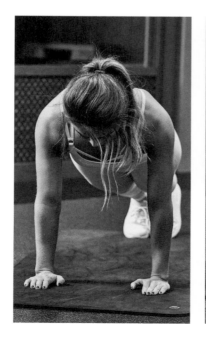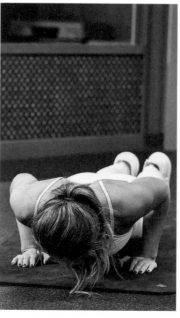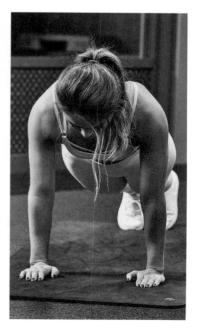

WORKOUTS

EXERCISE 2
DUMBBELL CHEST PRESS

EXERCISE 3
DUMBBELL FLIES

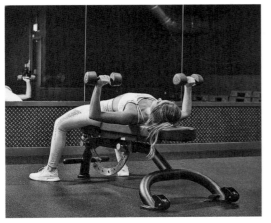

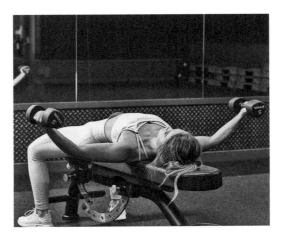

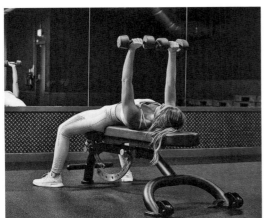

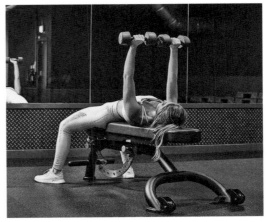

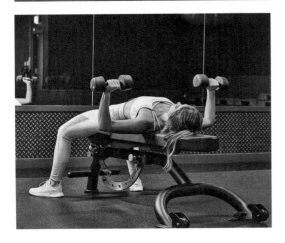

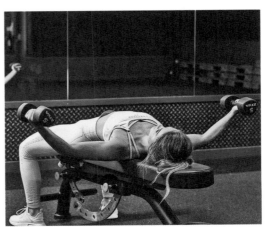

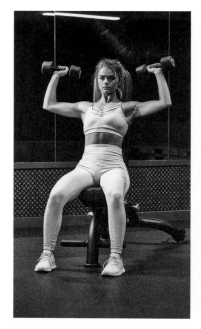 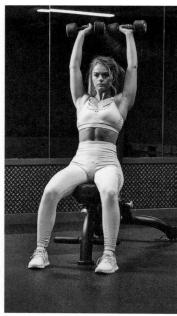 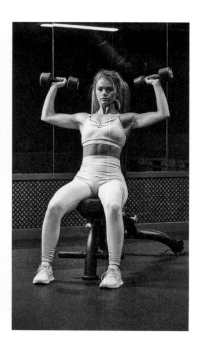

WIDE GRIP PUSH-UPS

The wide grip push-up is a really challenging exercise that
works your chest muscles hard.

EXERCISE 5
WIDE GRIP PUSH-UPS

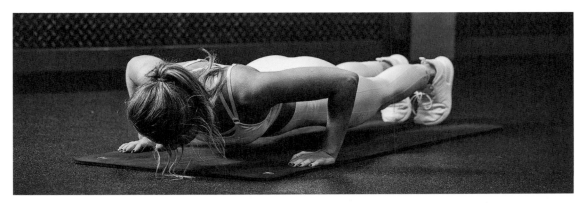

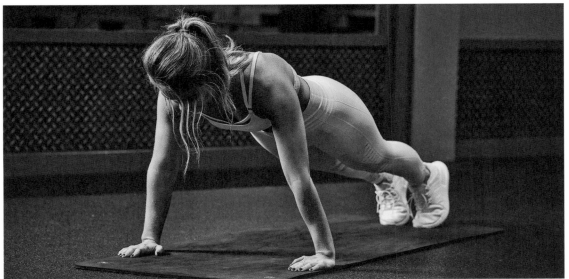

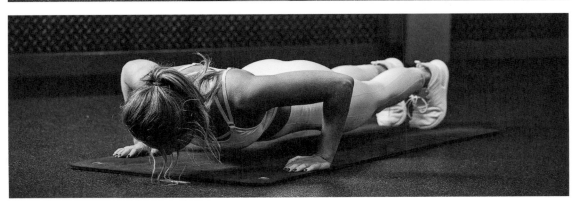

SHOULDERS, CHEST & TRICEPS
CIRCUIT 2

EXERCISE	TIME		
1	30 seconds	Seated lateral raises	
2	30 seconds	Plank to shoulder tap	
3	30 seconds	Dumbbell front raises	
4	30 seconds	Double arm tricep extensions	
5	30 seconds	Plank	

EXERCISE 1 – SEATED LATERAL RAISES

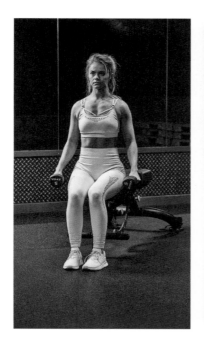 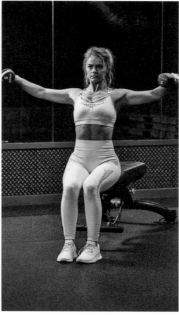 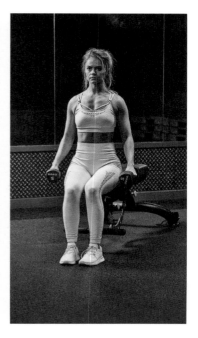

EXERCISE 2
PLANK TO SHOULDER TAP

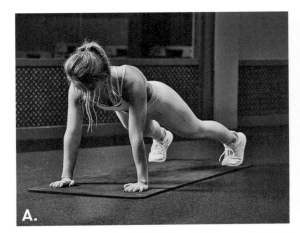

A.

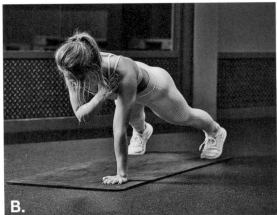

B.

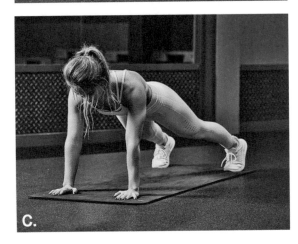

C.

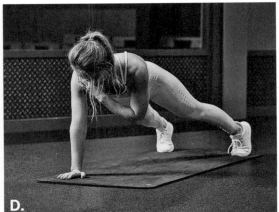

D.

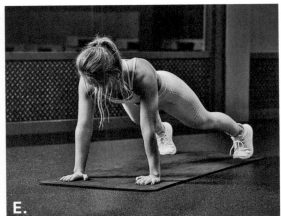

E.

EXERCISE 3 – DUMBBELL FRONT RAISES

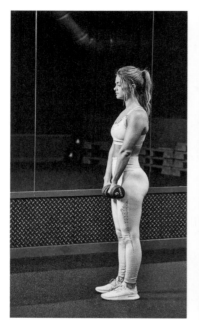
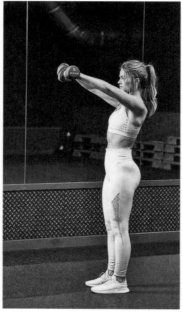
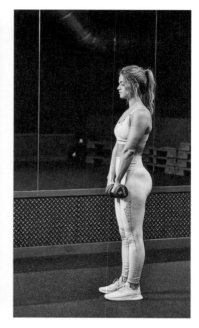

EXERCISE 4 – DOUBLE ARM TRICEP EXTENSIONS

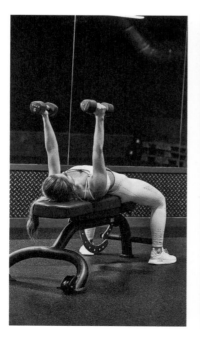
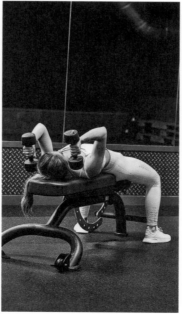
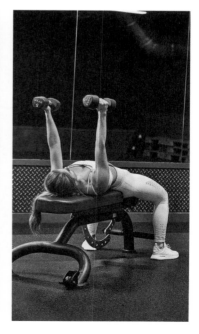

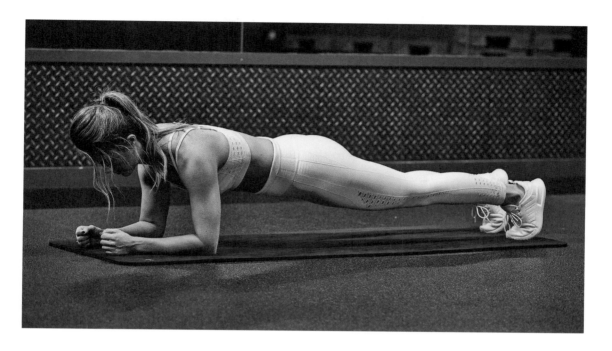

DUMBBELL FRONT RAISES . . .

. . . are perfect for working your front delts – essential for strong, sculpted shoulders. But don't go too heavy – by the 5th rep those dumbbells will feel much heavier than on the 1st.

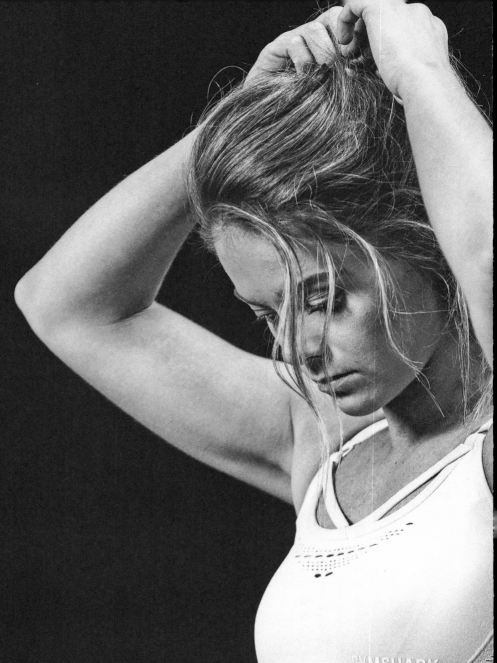

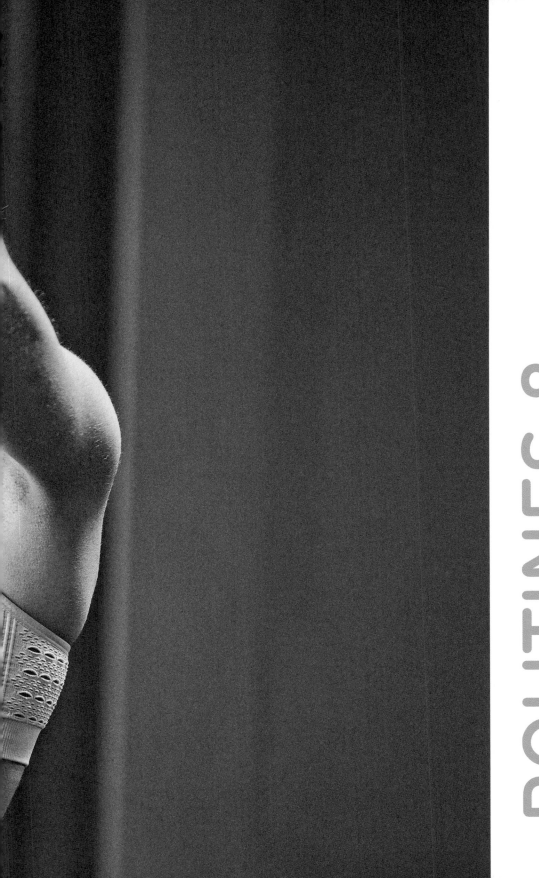

ROUTINES &
RITUALS

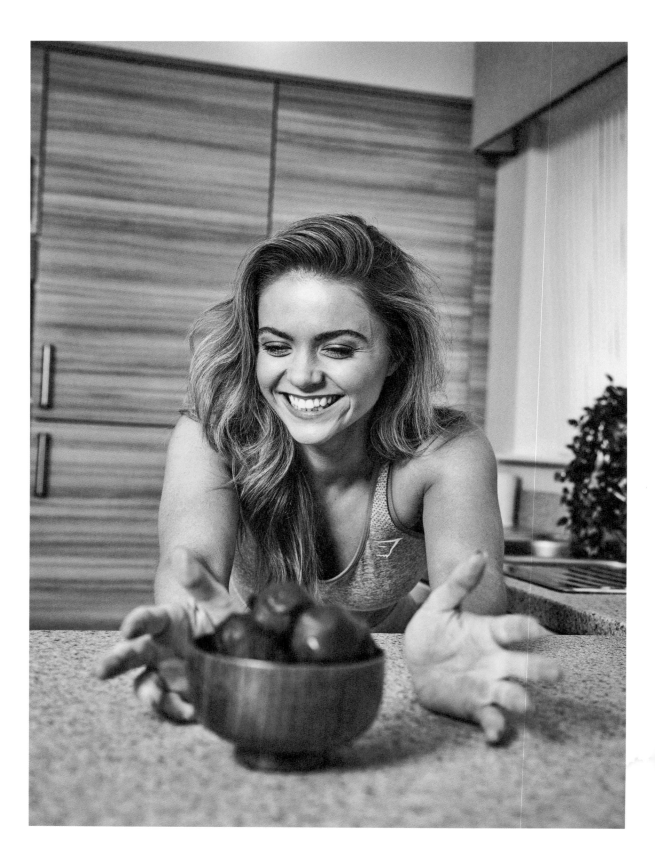

ROUTINES

PLANNING YOUR WEEK

Now that you have chosen your preferred workout plan for the week, let's talk about how to pair this with a meal plan to have the ultimate weekly schedule to take you closer to a stronger, healthier you. You can use the recipes in this book however you like, but it is always helpful to see what recipes are good for pre- or post-workouts, and what recipes work best for planning the week ahead.

The following weekly schedule is just one of many examples of how you can combine recipes and workouts – you can mix it up and pick and choose your favourite meals to add to your routine depending on your preferences. Having a set plan will allow you to see your week ahead, prepare and plan your grocery shopping and know what days you are committing to exercise. Having a plan is so important in being able to actually execute and stick to your goals.

So, grab a journal or a wall calendar and create a visual plan of what your week looks like. This way you can tick off your achievements as you go and reward yourself at the end of the week with your favourite self-care activity.

	MONDAY	TUESDAY	WEDNESDAY
BREAKFAST	Mango and ginger smoothie (page 22)	Almond butter and jam porridge (page 30)	Turmeric tofu scramble (page 38)
LUNCH	Deconstructed burrito bowl (page 61)	Lentil Bolognese (page 95)	Kung pao buddha bowl (page 58)
DINNER	Spiced carrot and lentil soup (page 51)	Lemon tofu flatbread with herb yogurt (page 110)	Mexican bean chilli (page 89)
SNACK	Vanilla and coconut protein ball (page 137)	Vanilla and coconut protein ball	Vanilla and coconut protein ball
WORKOUT	Day 1 Gym workout or Day 1 Home workout	Rest day or activity of your choice	DAY 2 Gym workout or Day 2 Home workout

A NOTE ON SNACKS

In this weekly plan, I've used vanilla and coconut protein balls as the suggested snack. The recipe makes 8 servings, so they're perfect to make at the beginning of the week and keep in the fridge. The same goes for my protein bars, muffins and trail mix bars – all handy to make in advance so you've got a healthy snack available at all times.

THURSDAY	FRIDAY	SATURDAY	SUNDAY
Chocolate lovers smoothie (page 20)	Blueberry and lemon pancakes (page 28)	Sweet potato and tempeh hash (page 47)	The ultimate British breakfast (page 40)
Mexican bean chilli (page 89)	Black bean and avocado breakfast wrap (page 43)	Summer rolls salad bowl (page 65)	Peanut butter buddha bowl (page 57)
Tofu Pad Thai (page 109)	Sesame orange seitan stir fry (page 80)	Chipotle black bean burgers (page 72)	Spiced carrot and lentil soup (page 51)
Vanilla and coconut protein ball	Vanilla and coconut protein ball	Beat it juice (page 25)	Post workout hulk juice (page 25)
Rest day or activity of your choice	DAY 3 Gym workout or Day 3 Home workout	DAY 4 Gym workout or Day 4 Home workout	Rest day

A NOTE ON LEFTOVERS

All the recipes in *Naturally Stefanie* can be doubled and kept in the fridge or freezer to eat as leftovers for your lunch or dinner during the week. On Wednesday, for example, I've suggested Mexican bean chilli for dinner and then eating the leftovers for Thursday's lunch. Making the most of leftovers really helps me to eat well. It also means I don't have to cook every day!

TIPS FOR HEALTHY EATING

1. 'FAILING TO PREPARE IS PREPARING TO FAIL'

Set out your meal plan for the week ahead, go grocery shopping and make sure you have everything you need. Many of the meals in the sample meal plan can be made in bulk or at least enough for two days, so if you know you are going to be busy and have limited time to make lunch, make it the day before. If you are making dinner anyway, you can just double up.

2. IF YOU BUY HEALTHY FOOD, YOU WILL EAT HEALTHY FOOD.

Sure, have a secret chocolate stash like me and have a square or two when you need it, but try for the most part to keep most of the food in your house healthy and make homemade sweets and snacks to curb cravings.

3. DRINK WATER AND STAY HYDRATED!

Try to reduce fizzy drinks and alcohol throughout the week and focus on hitting a water goal of 2 litres a day. Try setting an alarm to go off every hour to remind you to drink a glass of water – this is an easy way to achieve to the 2-litre goal.

4. EAT WHEN YOU ARE HUNGRY AND STOP WHEN YOU ARE FULL

It sounds straightforward but some of the recipes in this book might be larger portion sizes than you are used to. Don't force yourself to eat the whole batch if you can only eat half – listen to your body and its needs. This will be different for everyone!

5. ENJOY YOUR FOOD!

Food can be so much fun, experiment in the kitchen and get to know what you like. Make the recipes in this book for your friends and family; dinner parties are my favourite. Don't forget food is a social event, so don't restrict yourself – it's great to go out for an indulgent meal every now and then with friends.

RITUALS

A WELL-EARNED REST

Sleep is incredibly important for your body to rest and also to grow and repair. Your work in the gym actually breaks down your muscles, the food then helps them to heal and sleep allows them to build and grow.

Do. Not. Underestimate. Sleep.

Make sure after all of your hard work on eating healthily, working out and taking care of yourself that you prioritise at least 7 to 8 hours of sleep a night.

1. DRINK HERBAL TEA

I am a sucker for both peppermint and chamomile tea – I need a good three mugs a day – but I save chamomile for my pre-bed, night-time read to help me nod off to sleep.

2. PUT YOUR PHONE AWAY

I know it's been said many times before, but it's true that being on your phone will stimulate your brain – even if you are just aimlessly scrolling – tricking it into staying alert even if you are tired. Set your alarm, or better yet buy an alarm clock so your phone doesn't even need to be in your room, and read a book or listen to an audiobook before you settle down to sleep.

3. TAKE A BATH

Back to the self-love, a bath before bed is a game changer. Add some salts and lavender and soak away. Just try not to fall asleep in the bath. That is not advised.

4. WRITE DOWN YOUR GOALS

If I have 101 things running through my head of what I need to get done the next day, I will not sleep. I always write a to-do list for the next day before I go to bed, so it is on paper and out of my head. It will also help you to begin the next day feeling prepared and organised so you can start your new day as well as you ended the previous one.

5. ESTABLISH A NIGHT-TIME ROUTINE

Nothing fancy, just try to go to bed roughly the same time every night. I aim to be in bed by 10 p.m. and lights out by 11 p.m. at the latest. I am a sleep lover, so going to bed any later than that and then trying to wake up at 7 a.m. is not going to be beneficial for me; or anyone around me for that matter! Going to bed at the same time will train your body into knowing when to sleep and when to wake up – you will naturally start to feel tired at the same time every evening and your sleep will improve.

SELF-LOVE

> 'You can drink your water, eat your vegetables and do your exercise, but if you don't deal with what is going on in your head and your heart you will still be unhealthy.'

I truly believe in self-love and taking care of yourself in all aspects of your life. We live in such a busy and stressful world that it is important to take time out every now and then to take care of ourselves. This doesn't have to be anything drastic; I am not asking you to go on an all-inclusive yoga retreat in the Maldives. For you, this may be ten minutes a day of meditation, it may be a nightly bubble bath, a weekly face mask, Sunday mornings in bed with a book or a film; whatever it is, make time for it.

I want to share with you some of my top tips to making you feel positive, happy and confident in yourself and your body through some easy self-love practices you can do every week.

1. SKINCARE ROUTINE

Whether it's a bubble bath, face mask or even a spa day; whatever it is that makes you feel good about yourself, schedule time to do it! I personally have a bath once a week (don't worry, I shower on the other six days) and I take bath time very seriously. Bath time is me time. I run a bath, fill it with bubbles and one bath bomb too many, apply a face mask; usually over generously, get a bowl of ice cream and pop Netflix on my laptop in the corner. If that isn't next level self-love, I don't know what is.

2. CHOOSE HOW YOU SPEND YOUR TIME ONLINE

Social media has a bad reputation, especially when it comes to mental wellbeing. With this in mind, it is important to choose how you interact online, how much time you spend on social media and to decide if it really brings you happiness. I recommend seeing the positive sides of social media – use it for inspiration, motivation, and for following those who post positive and helpful content. Rid your feed of those who are negative and who aren't serving you any positive purpose. Perhaps be more of aware of when and how much you're using your phone – and pay attention to what might make you feel positive or negative online.

I started using social media to share my health and fitness journey in the hopes it would help at least someone else out there who needed it. If you use social media, you can consciously decide how you would like to use it to bring you and others happiness and inspiration. Remember, you are also only a click away from bringing positive people into your life online.

3. DO THINGS THAT MAKE YOU HAPPY

It is so important to focus on the good in your life! Focus on the things you have rather than those that you don't. Be grateful for your family and friends, be grateful for your health. This gratitude can also be applied to exercise: be thankful you have a body that is healthy and able to exercise, rather than hating it for not looking exactly the way you want it to. For me spending time with family and friends is what makes me happy, so I make sure I do that at least once a week. I usually go for walks with my best friend, make cake with my sister and visit my gran's on a Friday afternoon when all my aunts and cousins are in. Take the time to do the things that make you happy.

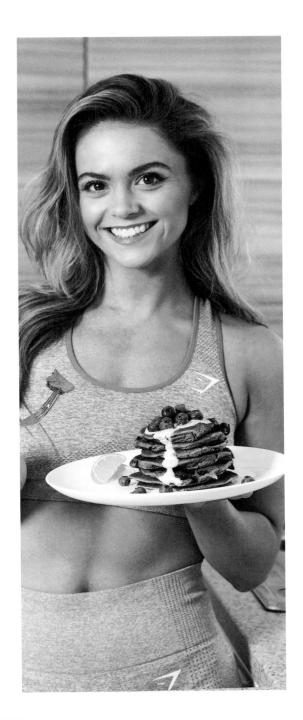

COOL DOWN

Thank you to all of you for reading this book. I hope it has inspired you to make some healthy lifestyle changes to your routine and that it will help you on your way to being a stronger, happier you. I want to round off with a final note on the top five things I hope you take away from *Naturally Stefanie*.

1. KEEP IT SIMPLE

Food should be easy and fun to make. There is no need to over complicate nutrition. Instead, make the simple healthy recipes in this book and say goodbye to fad diets.

2. PLAN AHEAD

Pick your meals for the week and stock up on all of the ingredients. That way you will be prepared and more likely to stick to your healthy meal choices.

3. BE REALISTIC

Find a workout routine that suits you. Whether you want to use the home or gym workouts in this book or a mix of the two, make a realistic weekly schedule that works for you and your lifestyle.

4. RELAX

Find downtime at least once a week. Self-care is so important in all areas of life so don't forget to unwind and relax at the end of a busy week.

5. HAVE FUN!

This is the most important take-away of all. I firmly believe in having a positive mental attitude (PMA), enjoying life and not taking anything too seriously. You live once, so eat your vegetables, kick butt in the gym, put on a face mask and don't forget to treat yourself with your chocolate stash.

ROUTINES & RITUALS

THANK YOU

I am so grateful to the people in my life who have made this book possible – from close family to new friends – I am thankful to you all.

First of all, thank you to the team over at Summer who have managed me for just over a year now. Your impact on my business has been amazing and I am so grateful for all of the opportunities you bring to me. I have met with quite a few management agencies over the years and no one was right to bring my crazy dreams and ideas to life. Special thanks to Bex, Katie and Sally Anne.

Thank you to the amazing publishers over at Black & White Publishing for believing in my ideas for this book and bringing them to life. Alice, you have been a dream. I knew as soon as we met in Edinburgh that you guys were the team for me and the *Naturally Stefanie* book. Thank you to Euan, our wonderful photographer, for putting up with my styling preferences and being patient with me spending 45 minutes trying to get that perfect burger shot!

My family are of course the centre of my life and thus, as you will have seen, they have made their fair share of appearances in this book. I have dedicated *Naturally Stefanie* to my parents; the two most important people in my life who have always supported everything I do – even when I quit the 9 to 5 world and started working on my own projects at the age of 22. To my gorgeous sister Sarah, my sidekick, my best friend – I am so proud to call you my sister and so proud of everything you have achieved. Thank you for always supporting me and my crazy ideas.

Marco, my other best friend and my husband. We had barely met when I decided to go vegan, start up my own business and made you my designated food tester. Thank you for always being by my side and I apologise in retrospect for the past food failures you had to endure. I love you for loving me enough to try them!

Finally, thank you to each and every person who has followed me on this journey so far. Without your constant support and love I would not be where I am today, and this book would not have been possible. I hope *Naturally Stefanie* brings more love and positivity to your life and we can have many more memories in this life together.

ABOUT STEFANIE MOIR

Stefanie Moir is a Top 5 Scottish social media influencer based in Glasgow. Stefanie is a vegan and fitness enthusiast who gained online popularity for her lifestyle channel, NaturallyStefanie. She is best known for sharing her gym routines and healthy vegan recipes, which have garnered her over 200,000 YouTube subscribers, and growing. Stefanie has over 313,000 followers on Instagram, and also runs vegan fitness site veganaesthetics.co.uk, where she provides seasonal 12-week programmes to thousands of members worldwide.

@naturallystefanie

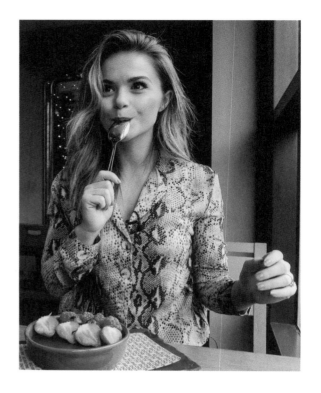